Emma Deslarzes

Cancer in Pets

Early Detection, Causes, Modern Therapies

bup

Emma Deslarzes
Cancer in Pets
Early Detection, Causes, Modern Therapies

ISBN: 978-3-69035-774-6

Order number: 2026-1
Also as an eBook
(978-3-69035-779-1)

Cover design: Kerstin Laube
Production: Angelika Haase

Copyright: Bremen University Press, 2025.
Fahrenheitstr. 11, 28359 Bremen
bup@bremenuniversitypress.com
www.bremenuniversitypress.com

The manuscript may not be used in whole or in part without the prior written consent of the publisher.

This book was printed on environmentally friendly paper from sustainable forestry in order to conserve resources and minimise environmental impact. By using recycled materials and FSC-certified paper, we are helping to protect forests and reduce our ecological footprint.

Emma Deslarzes

Cancer in Pets

Early Detection, Causes, Modern Therapies

Overview

PRELIMINARY REMARK		11
1.	INTRODUCTION	13
2.	BASICS OF TUMOUR BIOLOGY IN PETS	19
3.	EPIDEMIOLOGY AND RISK FACTORS	33
4.	CLINICAL SYMPTOMS AND PROGRESSION OF CANCER	47
5.	DIAGNOSTIC PROCEDURES IN VETERINARY ONCOLOGY	60
6.	CLASSIFICATION AND STAGING OF TUMOURS	74
7.	THERAPEUTIC APPROACHES AND HEALING METHODS	88
8.	QUALITY OF LIFE, CARE AND ETHICAL CONSIDERATIONS	107
9.	PREVENTION AND HEALTH CARE	114
10.	RESEARCH AND FUTURE PROSPECTS IN VETERINARY ONCOLOGY	125
11.	LEGAL AND INSURANCE-RELATED FRAMEWORK CONDITIONS	135
12.	FUTURE PROSPECTS AND NEW TREATMENT METHODS	142
13.	CONCLUDING REMARKS	146

14. BIBLIOGRAPHY **149**

Table of contents

PRELIMINARY REMARK		11
1.	**INTRODUCTION**	13
1.1	Definition: Cancer in pets - veterinary and biological perspectives	13
1.2	Significance of cancers in the veterinary context	14
1.3	Increase in oncological diseases in pets in a changing society	15
1.4	Objective	17
2.	**BASICS OF TUMOUR BIOLOGY IN PETS**	19
2.1	Cellular and molecular basis of tumour development	19
2.2	Different types of tumours in dogs and cats	22
2.3	Genetic, epigenetic and hormonal influences	26
2.4	Differences to human medical oncology	29
3.	**EPIDEMIOLOGY AND RISK FACTORS**	33
3.1	Prevalence and incidence in small animal practice	33
3.2	Race-related dispositions and genetic risks	35
3.3	Environmental factors, nutrition and postural influences	39
3.4	Age-related aspects and hormonal status changes	42
4.	**CLINICAL SYMPTOMS AND PROGRESSION OF CANCER**	47
4.1	Early detection and key clinical symptoms	47
4.2	Organ-related manifestations and atypical courses	50
4.3	Differences in symptoms between dogs and cats	53
4.4	Behaviour and pain as diagnostic indicators	56

5.	**DIAGNOSTIC PROCEDURES IN VETERINARY ONCOLOGY**	**60**
5.1	General veterinary examination techniques	60
5.2	Imaging procedures: X-ray, ultrasound, CT and MRI	62
5.3	Cytological and histopathological methods	65
5.4	Tumour markers, genetic tests and laboratory diagnostics	68
5.5	The role of telemedicine in the diagnosis of cancer in pets	71
6.	**CLASSIFICATION AND STAGING OF TUMOURS**	**74**
6.1	TNM system in veterinary medicine	74
6.2	Grading and histology of tumours	77
6.3	Relevance of staging for treatment decisions	80
6.4	Prognosis assessment and individual progression expectation	83
7.	**THERAPEUTIC APPROACHES AND HEALING METHODS**	**88**
7.1	Surgical forms of therapy and their limitations	88
7.2	Radiotherapy in small animal oncology	92
7.3	Chemotherapy: protocols, active substances and side effects	95
7.4	Immunotherapy, targeted therapy and personalised approaches	99
7.5	Stem cell-based therapies and regenerative medicine	102
7.6	Alternative medical methods and their scientific evaluation	105
7.7	Palliative medical measures for non-curative cases	106
8.	**QUALITY OF LIFE, CARE AND ETHICAL CONSIDERATIONS**	**107**
8.1	Quality of life assessment from a veterinary point of view	107
8.2	Communication between vet, pet owner and, if necessary, psychologist	110

8.3	Ethical aspects of the treatment decision	111
8.4	Hospice care and end-of-life care for animals	112
9.	**PREVENTION AND HEALTH CARE**	**114**
9.1	Vaccinations, castration and check-ups	114
9.2	Diet, exercise and avoidance of risk factors	117
9.3	Genetic screening in breeding animals	121
9.4	Education and training of animal owners	124
10.	**RESEARCH AND FUTURE PROSPECTS IN VETERINARY ONCOLOGY**	**125**
10.1	Current study situation and translational research status	125
10.2	Integration of AI, big data and molecular diagnostics	129
10.3	Development of innovative therapeutic approaches	130
10.4	Interdisciplinary collaboration with human medicine	133
11.	**LEGAL AND INSURANCE-RELATED FRAMEWORK CONDITIONS**	**135**
11.1	Liability issues in connection with diagnostics and therapy	135
11.2	Role of veterinary health insurance for oncological diseases	138
11.3	Duty to inform and consent of the holder	140
11.4	Documentation and reporting obligations for certain tumours	140
12.	**FUTURE PROSPECTS AND NEW TREATMENT METHODS**	**142**
13.	**CONCLUDING REMARKS**	**146**
14.	**BIBLIOGRAPHY**	**149**

9

Notes

- This book has a modular structure so that each chapter can be read independently without necessarily having to refer back to others.
- Processing status: March 2025

The publisher

Preliminary remark

The diagnosis of cancer is a word that is associated with fear, uncertainty and pain - not only in human medicine, but also in everyday veterinary practice. When a pet that is part of the family suffers from a tumour, vets and owners alike are faced with difficult decisions, medical challenges and emotional borderline situations. The treatment of oncological diseases in pets is no longer a marginal issue - it is now an integral part of modern small animal medicine and a reflection of our changing understanding of animal health, responsibility and care.

This book was written out of the conviction that oncology in veterinary medicine is not only advanced by technological progress and therapeutic innovations, but also by knowledge, education, ethical reflection and empathy. It is not intended to be a mere reference work, but a systematic and at the same time in-depth examination of all aspects of cancer in pets - from the biological basis and clinical practice to the question of what a dignified life and a responsible farewell can mean.

The structure of this work follows an interdisciplinary understanding of veterinary oncology: it combines molecular findings with clinical experience, sheds light on diagnostics and therapy as well as prevention, care and future prospects. The book is deliberately not aimed exclusively at veterinary specialists, but also at interested pet owners who are confronted with a cancer diagnosis and are looking for reliable, differentiated guidance.

At the same time, this book sees itself as a bridge between science and practice. It is intended to help people make informed decisions, strengthen their confidence in therapeutic processes and, not least, take the emotional complexity of cancer treatment in pets seriously. Because every medical decision is also a human one - based on love for the animal, respect for its life and the pursuit of a medicine that is more than the mere application of technical means.

I would like to thank all veterinarians, researchers and carers who advocate for the lives of our pets every day with expertise and compassion. I would also like to thank the pet owners who are prepared to stand by their animals with courage, patience and dedication, even when the going gets tough.

This book is dedicated to them all.

1. Introduction

1.1 Definition: Cancer in pets - veterinary and biological perspectives

The diagnosis of cancer in a pet is a particular challenge for pet owners and veterinarians alike. Cancer, medically known as malignant neoplasia, is an increasingly common disease in pets - especially dogs and cats - and has become more important in veterinary medicine in recent decades. There are many reasons for this, ranging from improved diagnostics and increased life expectancy of animals to environmental factors and breed-specific predispositions.

Dealing with this topic requires a sound knowledge of biological, diagnostic, therapeutic and ethical dimensions in order to provide the affected animals with appropriate treatment and animal owners with understandable, comprehensible support.

The term "cancer in pets" is used in this work to subsume all malignant tumour diseases that are of clinical relevance in veterinary practice. The veterinary perspective differs in many respects from human medical oncology, for example with regard to diagnostic strategies, therapeutic decision-making processes and the treatment of patients who are unable to express their symptoms verbally. This requires a particularly careful, attentive and structured approach, which requires both veterinary expertise and empathy towards the animal and its owner. At the same time, the subject requires an intensive examination of the biological basis of tumour development, epidemiological observations, technological advances in diagnostics and therapy as well as social developments that are changing the relationship between humans and animals.

1.2   Significance of cancers in the veterinary context

Cancer in pets is not only a medical problem, but also an emotionally and socially charged process that is accompanied by uncertainty, hope, powerlessness and decision-making difficulties. The role of the pet as a family member is increasingly coming to the fore, which has also changed the expectations of veterinary care. Whereas in earlier decades a cancer diagnosis often meant the inevitable end, today there is a broad spectrum of therapeutic options available, ranging from surgical interventions and radiotherapy to , drug treatment and palliative care. In modern veterinary medicine, it is therefore essential not only to combat the tumour itself, but also to maintain the quality of life of the affected animal and to involve the owners responsibly in the decision-making process.

1.3 Increase in oncological diseases in pets in a changing society

It is now well documented that cancers in dogs and cats are diagnosed more frequently than they were a few decades ago. However, this development is not solely due to an actual increase in tumour formation, but to a combination of several factors, some of which are biological, others technical or environmental in nature. One of the most important reasons is the significantly increased life expectancy of many pets. Thanks to advances in veterinary care, improved nutrition, consistent preventative measures and an increased awareness of health changes among owners, many dogs and cats are now reaching an age that was previously rare. As the majority of cancers occur at an older age, the longer lifespan inevitably means that the likelihood of tumours occurring also increases.

In addition, veterinary diagnostics have developed considerably. Modern imaging techniques such as computer tomography or magnetic resonance imaging, molecular biological diagnoses, fine needle biopsies and more comprehensive laboratory medical options make it easier than ever to detect even smaller or deeper tumours at an early stage. Many tumours that would have simply gone undetected in the past are now diagnosed, documented and treated. Statistically speaking, this leads to an apparent increase, even if part of this is due to a higher detection rate.

In addition to these medical-technical factors, changes in the environment also play a role. Increasing exposure to environmental toxins, pesticides, particulate matter, car exhaust fumes and tobacco smoke has not only contributed to an increase in cell-damaging processes in humans, but also in pets. Studies have shown that cats living in smoking households have a significantly increased risk of certain types of tumours. Dogs that are regularly walked on contaminated soils or in areas with heavy traffic are also exposed to increased risk factors. In addition, the lifestyle of many pets is becoming increasingly similar to that of humans: Lack of exercise, obesity, hormonal imbalances and constant contact with synthetic substances or highly processed feed can also favour cancer-causing processes.

Another aspect is genetic predisposition. In the course of the increasing pure breeding of certain dog breeds, hereditary diseases, including a genetic susceptibility to certain types of tumours, have also become more common. Particularly in large or highly selected breeds such as the Boxer, Rottweiler or St Bernard, there are clusters of certain cancers. There are also indications of a genetically determined increased susceptibility to tumours in cats, for example in certain lines of Siamese cats or in long-haired breeds.

Last but not least, the change in the perception of animals as family members also plays a role. Many pet owners today are prepared to take advantage of extensive diagnostics and therapies, even for older or chronically ill animals. This not only increases survival times, but also contributes to diseases such as cancer being recognised and documented more frequently. The increased attention therefore leads to an improved data basis, which epidemiologically results in an accumulation, even if the biological cancer risk may not have increased significantly in absolute figures.

1.4 Objective

The aim of this book is to provide a comprehensive presentation of the current state of knowledge on cancer in pets, covering biological, diagnostic and therapeutic aspects as well as ethical and emotional aspects. Special emphasis is placed on a comprehensible, yet precise and scientifically sound presentation, which is aimed at both readers with a background in veterinary medicine and interested pet owners. The explanations are intended to help clarify the complex relationships between tumour biology, diagnostics, therapy options and the individual care of affected animals, taking into account current developments as well as proven clinical practices.

The structure of the book follows a systematic outline: after the basic introduction to tumour biology, the most important epidemiological factors and risk groups in pets are presented. This is followed by detailed chapters on clinical symptoms, modern diagnostic procedures, staging and classification of tumours and the wide range of therapeutic measures available to veterinary medicine today. Particular attention is also paid to questions of quality of life, ethical decision-making and the care of pet owners in stressful situations. Finally, current research approaches and future perspectives will be discussed in order to provide an outlook on possible advances in veterinary oncological care.

The aim is to create a work that not only serves as a reference work, but also provides a deeper understanding of the complex reality of cancer in pets and contributes to the improvement of veterinary practice.

2. Basics of tumour biology in pets

2.1 Cellular and molecular basis of tumour development

Tumour biology is a central element in the understanding of oncological processes, not only in human medicine, but increasingly also in veterinary medicine. It provides the essential basis for understanding how cancers develop, how they develop and spread in the organism and how therapeutic interventions can be applied. Understanding these biological processes not only allows a sound clinical assessment, but also opens up perspectives for targeted, individualised treatment strategies. Particularly in veterinary oncology, which has made considerable progress in recent years, the study of the molecular pathogenesis of tumours is essential in order to treat pets with malignant diseases not only symptomatically, but also causally and effectively in the long term. In this respect, it has been shown that many principles of tumour development, growth and metastasis are largely identical in animals and humans, which makes it easier to transfer human medical research results to veterinary medicine. At the same time, however, there are species-specific differences in cell biology, the immune response and the pharmacokinetic reaction to therapeutic agents, which require a differentiated approach.

The start of a tumour process is always to be found in the derailment of cell division. In healthy tissues, the cell cycle is strictly controlled by a multitude of complex regulatory mechanisms. These mechanisms monitor every phase of cell division, from DNA replication to mitosis and cell division, and decide whether a cell is allowed to divide, whether it enters a dormant stage or whether it eliminates itself in a controlled manner through apoptosis. The integrity of these control mechanisms is crucial for tissue homeostasis, i.e. for the balance between new cell formation, differentiation and cell death. However, if there are disruptions in one or more of these checkpoints, a cell can escape physiological regulation. Such disturbances can be due to a variety of different causes. Particularly relevant are genetic mutations that either occur spontaneously or are induced by exogenous noxious agents such as radiation, chemical carcinogens or certain viruses. Epigenetic changes, i.e. reversible modifications of gene expression without changing the DNA sequence, can also contribute to an inhibition of the cell cycle.

Once initiated, the affected cell begins to divide independently of the normal regulatory signals. This leads to the formation of a clonally expanding cell cluster whose cells are genetically identical and often aggressively altered in their biological characteristics. The resulting tumour masses can vary greatly in their biological behaviour. Benign tumours usually grow slowly, show no invasion of the surrounding tissue and do not form metastases. They can, however, cause considerable clinical problems due to space requirements, pressure on neighbouring structures or hormonal activity. Malignant tumours, on the other hand, are characterised by uncontrolled, infiltrating growth, destruction of the surrounding tissue and the ability to spread to other parts of the body via blood or lymph channels and form metastases.

The ability to metastasise is a key feature of malignant tumours and represents one of the greatest therapeutic challenges. It requires individual tumour cells to lose cell adhesion, detach from the primary tumour, invade blood vessels, survive in the circulation, adhere to distant organs and proliferate there again. Each of these phases is controlled by specific molecular mechanisms that are being intensively studied in modern tumour research. The aim is to identify the signalling pathways that are responsible for the invasive and metastatic behaviour of tumour cells in order to develop targeted pharmacological interventions that can inhibit these processes.

Another key element in tumour biology is the tumour microenvironment. Tumour cells are not isolated in the tissue, but are in constant interaction with their environment, i.e. with connective tissue cells, immune cells, vessels and the extracellular matrix. This environment can significantly influence the growth and therapy resistance of tumours. For example, tumour cells can stimulate angiogenesis, i.e. the formation of new blood vessels, by releasing certain cytokines and growth factors in order to ensure their own supply of oxygen and nutrients. At the same time, they can suppress the host's immune response through immunomodulatory mechanisms, which enables them to survive virtually undisturbed.

In summary, tumour biology is a multi-layered, dynamic process that results from a complex interplay of genetic, epigenetic, cellular and environmental factors. For veterinary practice, this means that successful cancer therapy cannot be based on surgical or pharmacological measures alone, but requires an integrative approach based on a profound understanding of the biological principles . This is the only way to develop therapies that not only target tumour growth, but also its molecular causes and systemic consequences. This perspective is crucial in order to achieve a long-term improvement in the quality of life and survival time of pets suffering from cancer.

2.2   Different types of tumours in dogs and cats

The diversity of tumour diseases in dogs and cats is reflected in the variety of tissue types from which malignant or benign neoplasms can arise. A basic classification results from the assignment of the respective tumour to its tissue of origin. This differentiation is not only important for histological diagnosis, but also has a profound impact on therapeutic decision-making and the prognosis of the disease in question. Tumours differ considerably in their biological behaviour, their growth rate, their tendency to metastasise and their sensitivity to therapeutic measures - depending on whether they originate from epithelial, connective, muscle, blood or nerve tissue.

Epithelial tumours are among the most common neoplasms in pets. They develop from cells of the epithelial tissue that lines the outer skin as well as the inner and outer mucous membranes. This category includes squamous cell carcinomas, adenocarcinomas of the salivary glands, mammary gland carcinomas and tumours of the gastrointestinal tract. Epithelial tumours are often easy to differentiate and tend to metastasise to varying degrees, depending on the degree of differentiation and the type of tumour. In cats, adenocarcinomas of the mammary gland are particularly feared, as they generally have an aggressive biology and metastasise early. In dogs, on the other hand, benign epithelial neoplasms, such as benign adenomas, occur more frequently and are easily treatable by surgery. The treatment of epithelial tumours is often based on surgical removal in combination with adjuvant chemotherapy, although radiotherapy can also be used for certain localisations, such as in the head and neck area.

Mesenchymal tumours arise from the embryonic mesenchyme and therefore affect all tissues that develop from connective, bone, muscle, cartilage or fatty tissue. This group includes a variety of sarcomas, such as fibrosarcomas, haemangiosarcomas, osteosarcomas and liposarcomas. Mesenchymal tumours are often characterised by their infiltrative form of growth. They grow diffusely into the surrounding tissue and are therefore often difficult to remove completely. Their metastasis is also usually haematogenous, i.e. via the bloodstream, and typically manifests itself in the lungs or in parenchymal organs. Particularly in osteosarcoma in dogs, which occurs preferentially in the long tubular bones of larger breeds, systemic spread is likely at the time of initial diagnosis. The treatment of these tumours places high demands on surgical precision, often requires radical interventions such as amputations and in many cases is supplemented by chemotherapy to combat microscopic metastases.

Haematopoietic and lymphatic neoplasms are another important category of tumours. They include lymphomas (lymph nodes), leukaemias, plasmocytomas and other malignant changes in the haematopoietic system. In contrast to solid tumours, these diseases usually manifest themselves systemically, i.e. they affect several organs at the same time and often cannot be surgically removed. Lymphoma is one of the most common malignant diseases in dogs and can take various forms - from the highly malignant, rapidly progressive form to chronic subtypes with less aggressiveness. Alimentary lymphoma, which primarily affects the gastrointestinal tract, is particularly common in cats. Haematopoietic tumours are treated almost exclusively with medication. The combination of different cytostatic drugs according to standardised protocols can lead to a remission in many cases and significantly improve the quality of life of the animals. Nevertheless, the prognosis often depends on the stage of the disease, the cell line affected and the response to treatment.

In addition to these main categories, there are numerous other tumour types, such as neuroendocrine tumours, melanomas, mast cell tumours and tumours of the central nervous system, each of which has its own biological and therapeutic characteristics. Mast cell tumours in particular deserve attention in veterinary medicine, as they are one of the most common skin neoplasms in dogs and exhibit extremely variable biological behaviour. The entire spectrum is represented, from completely harmless, localised tumours to highly malignant, metastatic forms. Treatment can be surgical, medicinal or radiobiological, with molecular markers such as the Ki-67 proliferation index or c-kit mutations increasingly being used today for prognostic assessment.

Overall, it can be stated that the classification of tumours according to the tissue of origin not only serves the purpose of classification and nomenclature, but is also a fundamental tool for clinical decision-making. It allows a more precise prognosis assessment, differentiated therapy planning and is a prerequisite for the development of forward-looking, individualised treatment strategies. Knowledge of the different types of tumours in dogs and cats is therefore of fundamental importance not only for pathologists and oncologists, but for all veterinarians working in small animal medicine.

2.3 Genetic, epigenetic and hormonal influences

The genetic basis of tumour development in pets is increasingly becoming the focus of veterinary research, as it provides valuable insights into the molecular mechanisms underlying the development and progression of neoplasia. It is now well documented that numerous tumours in dogs and cats are triggered or at least facilitated by specific genetic changes. Particularly noteworthy are mutations in oncogenes, i.e. genes that promote cell growth when activated, and in tumour suppressor genes, whose function is to control the cell cycle and induce apoptosis. Equally important are defects in genes that are responsible for repairing DNA damage, as such defects favour the accumulation of mutations and can therefore promote tumour progression.

An impressive example of genetic predisposition is the observable breed-specific clustering of certain types of tumours. Osteosarcoma, for example, is more common than average in large dog breeds such as the Great Dane, the Rottweiler or the Irish Wolfhound. The high incidence of these aggressive bone tumours cannot be explained solely by biomechanical factors such as body weight, but also indicates a genetically anchored susceptibility that may have been unintentionally increased by targeted breeding. The same applies to mast cell tumours, which show a conspicuous accumulation in boxers. Here too, molecular genetic studies suggest that certain mutations, for example in the c-kit gene, play a central role in the development of tumours. Some of these genetic changes can now be detected by molecular diagnostics and open up new avenues for targeted therapies.

In addition to these firmly established genetic causes, epigenetic changes are becoming increasingly important in research into tumour biology. Unlike genetic mutations, epigenetic modifications do not change the sequence of the genetic material, but control gene activity through reversible biochemical processes. These include DNA methylation, in which methyl groups are attached to the DNA, thereby silencing genes, the modification of histone proteins, which regulate the packaging of DNA in the cell nucleus, and the expression of microRNAs, which can specifically inhibit the translation of certain mRNA molecules. These epigenetic processes react extremely sensitively to external stimuli and environmental factors, which makes them a key field in the question of how the environment and genetics interact in tumour development. In particular, influences such as chemical carcinogens, chronic inflammation, hormonal imbalances or malnutrition can permanently alter epigenetic patterns and thus contribute to the malignant transformation of cells. The reversibility of epigenetic modifications also makes them a promising therapeutic target, which is already the subject of intensive research in human medicine and is also increasingly finding its way into veterinary oncological research.

Another important aspect of genetic and epigenetic tumour biology concerns hormonally controlled tumours. Neoplasms of the mammary gland, testicles and thyroid gland are particularly relevant here. These tumour types are often closely linked to the hormonal balance of the organism and are dependent on hormonal stimuli for their growth and differentiation. For example, it is known that non-spayed bitches have a significantly increased risk of developing mammary tumours, whereby this connection is explained by the influence of female sex hormones on the epithelial tissue of the mammary gland. Hormonal influences also play a significant role in testicular tumours, which occur more frequently in cryptorchid males in particular. In thyroid tumours, on the other hand, a dysregulation of the hormonal feedback loops is often involved, which can lead to proliferative changes. In modern oncology, hormonal receptors on tumour cells are therefore increasingly being investigated in order to better understand the therapeutic potential of hormonal blockade or modulation and to be able to use it in a targeted manner.

Overall, it is clear that genetic predispositions, epigenetic control mechanisms and hormonal influences together form a complex network that determines the development and progression of tumour diseases in domestic animals. Deciphering this network is one of the major challenges in veterinary oncology and at the same time one of the most promising prospects for the development of new, individualised forms of diagnosis and therapy. A deeper understanding of these biological principles makes it possible to identify animals with an increased genetic risk at an early stage, take preventive measures, develop targeted therapies and thus substantially improve the prognosis of dogs and cats suffering from cancer.

2.4 Differences to human medical oncology

Compared to human medicine, tumour biology in domestic animals reveals a number of specific characteristics that are not only relevant from a clinical perspective, but also allow fundamental conclusions to be drawn about the interplay of genetics, environment and behaviour in the context of cancer development. One particularly striking feature is the different spontaneous incidence of certain tumour types between humans and animals. While some cancers are particularly common in humans, other forms are over-represented in dogs and cats, which points to species-specific biological characteristics as well as different environmental stresses, behavioural patterns and lifestyle habits. For example, mast cell tumours, lymphomas and osteosarcomas occur far more frequently in dogs than in humans, whereas liver and pancreatic carcinomas are rarer in comparison. In cats, on the other hand, alimentary lymphoma is particularly common, while other tumour forms such as thyroid carcinomas are relatively rare. These differences not only allow conclusions to be drawn about breed-specific genetic dispositions or exogenous risk factors, but also enable a targeted comparative analysis of disease progression, therapeutic responsiveness and molecular pathomechanisms.

An outstanding aspect of veterinary tumour research is the possibility of observing and analysing the natural course of disease in pets. In contrast to artificially induced tumour models in laboratory animal research, dogs and cats develop their tumour diseases spontaneously, i.e. under real conditions, which makes them particularly valuable models for comparative oncology. This discipline, which deals with the overlap between human and veterinary cancer research, is becoming increasingly important. In many translational studies today, pets, especially dogs, serve as a bridge between preclinical basic research and clinical application in humans. Due to their genetic diversity, their physiological similarity to human processes and their natural disease development, they offer a unique field of investigation for testing new therapeutic approaches, identifying biomarkers or better understanding immunological reactions in the course of oncological diseases. The experience gained in veterinary oncology not only flows into the care of animals, but also makes a valuable contribution to the further development of therapeutic approaches in human medicine.

Particularly noteworthy in this context is the increasing interest in innovative forms of therapy such as immunotherapy, which focuses on activating the body's own immune system to fight tumour cells. Initial studies on dogs with malignant melanomas or lymphomas have shown that certain immunomodulating strategies originally developed for humans can also be remarkably effective in animals. In addition, the efficacy and safety of new drugs is tested in pets before they are used in human clinical trials, which allows animals to participate in advanced therapeutic options at an early stage and at the same time increases the relevance of the results for human medicine.

For all these reasons, tumour biology in companion animals can be described as a dynamic, highly interdisciplinary field of research that combines clinical practice, molecular medicine, genetics, immunology and pharmacology. Its central aim is not only to improve individual veterinary care, but also to expand our understanding of carcinogenesis as an overall biological process. The investigation of cellular signalling pathways, genetic changes, epigenetic modifications and immunological interactions forms the basis for modern, personalised veterinary oncology that is tailored to the individual needs and biological conditions of each patient.

Understanding these processes is therefore not just a theoretical exercise, but also a practical tool that refines diagnostics, clarifies therapy and sustainably improves the quality of life of affected animals. At the same time, the close connection to human medicine offers the opportunity to utilise the findings of both disciplines synergistically and to shape the medicine of the future, in which the benefits for animals and humans are equally at the centre of attention. Tumour biology thus forms the indispensable foundation for all subsequent clinical, diagnostic and therapeutic considerations, which are presented in more detail below.

3. Epidemiology and risk factors

3.1 Prevalence and incidence in small animal practice

The epidemiological study of cancer in pets is an essential component of veterinary oncology, as it helps to recognise systematic patterns of disease distribution, identify risk factors and thus develop evidence-based preventive and therapeutic strategies. It deals with the frequency, geographical and demographic distribution and temporal development of oncological diseases in animal populations and thus forms a crucial interface between clinical practice, basic research and public health. Despite the fact that veterinary epidemiology does not have access to the same dense network of databases and register systems as human medicine, retrospective case analyses, veterinary register data, routine pathological data and clinical studies are providing increasingly reliable information on the spread and dynamics of tumour diseases in dogs and cats.

This shows that the prevalence and incidence of oncological diseases is significantly influenced by species-specific, breed-specific, gender-specific and age- and environment-dependent factors. Dogs are generally considered to be more affected by malignant neoplasia than cats, although there are considerable differences in tumour susceptibility within the species. The correlation between age and cancer risk is particularly striking. The probability of tumours in dogs increases significantly with age. Studies from the United States and Europe show that cancer is one of the most common causes of death in dogs over the age of ten and is responsible for around 45 per cent of deaths in older animals. Large and fast-growing breeds are particularly susceptible to certain types of tumours, such as osteosarcoma in Great Danes and haemangiosarcoma in Golden Retrievers.

Cancer is also a leading cause of death in cats, although the epidemiological patterns differ from those in dogs. Cats seem to develop benign tumours less frequently, which means that the presence of a mass is more often associated with a malignant change. This fact underlines the importance of early and comprehensive diagnosis in feline patients, especially as many feline tumours have an aggressive biology and become symptomatic late. Malignant lymphoma, squamous cell carcinoma - for example in the mucous membrane of the mouth - and adenocarcinomas of the mammary gland are particularly common in cats. The latter show a significantly higher malignancy rate compared to dogs in , which in turn speaks in favour of the importance of castration as a preventative measure, as hormonal influences have a significant impact on the risk of development.

In addition to biological factors, husbandry conditions, feeding behaviour, exposure to environmental toxins and access to veterinary care also play an important role in the epidemiological profile of oncological diseases. Studies show that animals that live in urban areas and are more frequently exposed to environmental pollution such as exhaust fumes or tobacco smoke have an increased risk of developing certain tumours. Chronic infections, for example with the feline leukaemia virus or the feline immunodeficiency virus, are also able to promote the development of malignant diseases such as lymphomas and therefore have both infectious-epidemiological and oncological relevance.

The findings from veterinary epidemiology are not only important for individual animals, but also for the further development of veterinary health care as a whole. They provide the basis for targeted prevention programmes, breeding strategies to reduce genetic risk factors and scientifically sound recommendations for the early detection of tumours. In addition, they enable an assessment of future trends, for example with regard to the influence of demographic change in the domestic animal population , increasing life expectancy or the impact of new environmental factors on the oncological disease spectrum.

3.2 Race-related dispositions and genetic risks

A particularly revealing epidemiological aspect in veterinary oncology is the breed-specific disposition, which can be observed as a significant accumulation of certain tumour diseases within specific dog breeds. These genetically determined susceptibilities are the result of complex selection processes within organised breeding and are based on the targeted reproduction of certain external characteristics, which are, however, often unintentionally linked to genetic risk factors for tumour diseases. The systematic recording of these predispositions not only provides valuable information for causal research, but also offers concrete starting points for individualised prevention, targeted early detection measures and breeding prevention strategies.

Such breed-specific predispositions are particularly evident in tumours of the haematopoietic system and mesenchymal tissue. Boxers, Labrador Retrievers and Golden Retrievers have an above-average incidence of mast cell tumours, with aggressive variants of this type of tumour occurring more frequently in these dog breeds. The biological characteristics of these tumours can range from slow-growing, benign skin changes to highly malignant, metastatic neoplasms, which makes regular clinical monitoring necessary, especially in predisposed animals. Sheepdogs, on the other hand, are particularly frequently affected by haemangiosarcomas, an aggressive form of tumour that primarily originates from the vascular endothelium and typically manifests itself in the spleen, liver or atrium. These tumours are characterised by a high risk of internal bleeding and are often only discovered when acute, life-threatening symptoms are already present.

The genetic predisposition is even more pronounced in osteosarcoma, which occurs preferentially in large and giant dog breeds such as the Great Dane, the Irish Wolfhound, the St Bernard or the Rottweiler. This type of tumour is known for its high aggressiveness, its rapid metastasis, particularly to the lungs, and its poor prognosis, even with early diagnosis and aggressive treatment. The particularly high susceptibility of these breeds to osteosarcoma cannot be explained solely by biomechanical stresses on large bone structures, but also points to a deeply rooted genetic predisposition that has hardly been addressed by breeding in recent decades.

Knowledge of these breed-specific risks is of great practical importance for veterinarians, as it enables more intensive monitoring within endangered populations and a more differentiated assessment of even subtle clinical changes. Early diagnostics, such as imaging techniques, cytology or histological analyses, can be used in a targeted manner to improve the prognosis and initiate treatment in good time. Furthermore, this also gives rise to an ethical and health policy responsibility on the part of breeding associations to take genetic risks seriously and minimise them through appropriate breeding control measures.

Certain tumour predispositions can also be found in cats, although the scientific data on this is much less extensive than in dogs. Studies suggest that Persian cats have an increased incidence of tumours in the nasopharynx, which may be related to their specific head shape, the so-called brachycephalic features. There is also a suspected genetic predisposition to malignant lymphomas in Siamese cats, although reliable long-term epidemiological data is still largely lacking. However, the evidence available to date is sufficient to sharpen clinical awareness in these breeds and to take early differential diagnostic action in suspected cases.

Vaccine-associated fibrosarcoma, a highly malignant soft tissue tumour associated with certain injection sites, also plays a particularly important role in feline oncology. This tumour usually occurs at sites where cats are routinely vaccinated - particularly in the neck or shoulder area - and was first systematically described in the 1990s. It is assumed that the chronic inflammatory reaction to the injection of certain adjuvants can promote a transformation of the surrounding connective tissue. Although the occurrence of this type of tumour is rare, it has led to far-reaching discussions in veterinary practice about the safety of vaccines, the selection of suitable injection sites and the need for alternative forms of application. It is now recommended that vaccines be administered into peripheral limbs or subcutaneously in the posterior thigh area where possible to facilitate complete surgical removal in the event of tumour growth.

Overall, the breed-specific disposition for tumour diseases in dogs and cats illustrates the great importance of genetic factors in the development of tumours and at the same time shows the potential of targeted preventive and control measures. The systematic collection and evaluation of such epidemiological patterns not only contributes to the improvement of individual veterinary care, but also to long-term health promotion within the populations themselves. It forms the basis for future-oriented breeding strategies, early diagnostic procedures and preventive veterinary medicine, which increasingly relies on genetic risk assessment and personalised care.

3.3 Environmental factors, nutrition and husbandry influences

In addition to genetic influences, environmental factors play a decisive role in the development of cancer in pets. Numerous observations and scientific studies indicate that certain external influences can significantly increase the risk of tumours developing. The affected animals are usually exposed to these influences over long periods of time without their owners being aware of the possible health consequences. The link between the environment and cancer is not limited to individual factors, but results from the complex interplay of various stresses that can reinforce each other.

There is a particularly clear link between exposure to harmful substances and the occurrence of certain types of cancer. Dogs that live in households with smokers not only passively inhale cigarette smoke, but also absorb the carcinogenic substances it contains through their skin and mucous membranes. The upper respiratory tract is particularly sensitive - nasal tumours have been described in long-nosed dogs and lung tumours in short-nosed breeds. Tobacco smoke also has an indirect negative effect on cats: They frequently groom their fur and in the process absorb pollutants that have been deposited there from the indoor air. These toxins enter the organism via the mucous membrane and can cause cell changes that contribute to the development of tumours. Other environmental toxins such as pesticides, solvents, flame retardants or certain household cleaners can also be absorbed through direct contact or through food and have carcinogenic effects. In some cases, repeated, low-dose exposure is enough to increase the risk in the long term.

Another environmental factor that is often underestimated is sun exposure. The risk of so-called UV-induced skin tumours is significantly increased, especially in cats with light or white coats that like to spend time outdoors regularly. Intense or repeated UV exposure can lead to the development of squamous cell carcinomas, especially on poorly furred areas of the body such as the edges of the ears, the nose or eyelids. These tumours are often inconspicuous in their early stages, but tend to spread into deeper layers of tissue if they are not treated. Direct exposure to the sun can also increase the risk of skin cancer in dogs with light-coloured skin or short, thin coats, especially if they are regularly kept in outdoor areas exposed to the south.

In addition to chemical and physical environmental factors, nutrition is increasingly becoming the focus of research as a potential cancer-promoting or cancer-protecting influence. Although the scientific data in veterinary medicine is not yet as comprehensive as in human medicine, there is increasing evidence that certain feed additives, preservatives or inadequately balanced diets could increase the risk of tumour diseases. An unbalanced diet, which leads to deficiency symptoms, can impair cell metabolism and weaken the defence against malignant cells. The connection between obesity and hormone-dependent tumours, such as mammary tumours in unspayed female dogs or prostate tumours in older male dogs, also appears to be particularly relevant. Being overweight not only changes the hormone balance, but also favours inflammatory processes in the body, which in turn are considered a risk factor for the development of certain types of cancer.

The way the animals live and are kept also has an influence on their individual cancer risk. Animals that are permanently kept indoors and receive little physical exercise are more prone to metabolic changes, obesity and a weakened immune system. A lack of physical activity affects hormone regulation, blood flow to the tissues and the function of the body's own repair mechanisms, among other things. At the same time, inadequate hygiene can increase the risk of chronic inflammation - for example in the area of the skin or mucous membranes - which in turn is considered a factor that favours malignant cell changes. Chronic inflammatory conditions lead to the constant formation of new cells, which increases the likelihood of errors in cell division and can therefore contribute to the development of tumours.

Overall, it is clear that the interactions between environment, behaviour and cell biology are extremely complex and cannot be reduced to individual factors. Rather, a holistic risk profile emerges, which consists of the sum of several small influences whose effects add up over the lifetime of the animal. For this reason, comprehensive prevention, which not only takes genetic dispositions into account, but also includes environmental conditions, diet, exercise and husbandry, is of crucial importance. Conscious design of the living environment, avoidance of known harmful substances, control of body weight and species-appropriate husbandry can make a significant contribution to reducing the risk of tumours in pets and at the same time improve their quality of life in the long term.

3.4 Age-related aspects and hormonal status changes

Another significant influencing factor in the development of cancer in pets is the hormonal constitution, i.e. the hormonal status of the respective animal. Hormones control a variety of biological processes, including the growth, maturation and renewal of tissues. These hormonal control mechanisms are essential for the normal functioning of the body, but can also contribute to the development of certain types of tumours if they are disrupted or excessive. This connection is particularly evident in hormone-dependent tumours, i.e. those whose growth is promoted by certain sex hormones such as oestrogen, progesterone or testosterone.

In bitches, the development of mammary tumours - i.e. tumours of the mammary glands - is closely linked to hormone levels. Studies show that non-spayed bitches have a significantly higher risk of developing such tumours in the course of their lives. This risk increases with each heat cycle, as the mammary glands are regularly under the influence of female sex hormones, which stimulate the tissue to change and grow. However, if a bitch is spayed before the first or second heat at the latest, the risk of mammary tumours is reduced to a fraction of the original value. This preventive effect of spaying is well documented medically and is often used in veterinary practice as an argument in favour of early spaying, provided that no breeding use is planned.

A similar correlation also exists in uncastrated male dogs, which have an increased risk of developing testicular tumours. Animals with so-called testicular retention, in which one or both testicles have not fully descended into the scrotum, are particularly affected. These testicles are then usually located in the abdominal cavity or in the inguinal canal, where the higher temperature compared to the scrotum tissue changes the cell structure and favours the development of tumours. There is also a connection between hormonal status and the development of certain tumours in older cats, particularly in the prostate or skin glands. Neutering can also help to reduce the risk of cancer in these cases, although the scientific data on this is less extensive for cats than for dogs.

The decision for or against castration should therefore not be made solely from the point of view of reproduction or behaviour control, but also with regard to the long-term health risk, particularly in the area of tumour prevention. In addition to the oncological aspects, the hormonal constitution also influences behaviour, metabolism, weight development and other health-relevant parameters, so that an individual assessment with the vet is advisable in each individual case.

Age is an equally important risk factor for the development of tumours. As dogs and cats get older, the likelihood of developing cancer increases significantly. This can be explained by several biological mechanisms. Firstly, external stresses - such as environmental toxins, radiation or infections - have a cumulative effect on the organism over a lifetime. This means that the longer an animal lives, the greater the probability that its cells will be exposed to harmful influences over time, which can cause mutations in the genetic material.

On the other hand, the internal cell processes also change with age. The ability of cells to recognise and repair DNA damage decreases. This leads to increasing instability of the genetic material, which forms the basis for uncontrolled cell division and therefore tumour growth. At the same time, the control of the cell cycle decreases, which means that faulty or degenerated cells are less reliably stopped or eliminated. The immune system, which normally plays an important role in recognising and eliminating tumour cells, also loses efficiency with age. This so-called immune senescence makes it more difficult for the body to defend itself against malignant cells, allowing them to multiply and spread unhindered.

All these processes mean that older animals have a significantly increased risk of cancer. For this reason, preventive care is particularly important for older dogs and cats. Regular veterinary examinations - ideally once a year or even more frequently if there are known risk factors - make it possible to recognise pathological changes at an early stage, even before they become clinically apparent. Modern diagnostic methods such as blood tests, imaging procedures and targeted tumour marker analyses help to detect even invisible or asymptomatic tumours in good time.

Early diagnosis improves the treatment options in many cases and can make a decisive contribution to the quality of life and prolongation of life of the affected animal. Oncological prevention in old age is therefore a central component of responsible pet ownership and should be just as much a matter of course as vaccinations, parasite control or dental care. With the increasing life expectancy of our pets - which is constantly rising thanks to improved medical care - this aspect will become even more important in the future.

4. Clinical symptoms and progression of cancer

4.1 Early detection and key clinical symptoms

The clinical symptoms of cancer in pets pose a particular diagnostic challenge because they vary greatly, are often non-specific and are often only clearly recognisable late in the course of the disease. Unlike humans, who can express pain or discomfort in words, veterinarians are dependent on carefully interpreting subtle physical or behavioural changes and placing them in a differentiated diagnostic context. This requires not only experience and attention on the part of the specialists, but also a high degree of sensitivity and observation on the part of the pet owners. This is because cancer often begins with small, seemingly insignificant changes in behaviour, food intake or physical activity that can easily be overlooked or misinterpreted.

A central element of early tumour detection is the knowledge of typical leading symptoms and organ manifestations, coupled with the awareness that the actual manifestation of the symptoms strongly depends on the location, size, growth dynamics and biological activity of the tumour. The most common visible or palpable signs include lumps, swellings or circumferential growths in the skin, subcutaneous tissue or in easily accessible areas of the body such as the groin, armpit or chest. These changes are usually characterised by a firm consistency, an irregular demarcation from the surrounding tissue and a slow but steady increase in size. Such tumours are often not painful in the early stages and initially have little effect on the animal's general condition, which means that they are either not noticed at all or are mistakenly classified as harmless skin changes, lipomas or cysts. However, the incidence of skin and subcutaneous tumours is particularly high in dogs, which makes their regular palpation as part of home care especially important.

Internal tumours, on the other hand, usually only manifest themselves in more advanced stages or when they impair the function of organs due to their size, location or infiltrating growth. For example, tumours of the gastrointestinal tract often only become clinically apparent when they lead to persistent digestive disorders, loss of appetite, chronic vomiting or weight loss. Abdominal tumours, for example on the liver, spleen or pancreas, can cause acute symptoms due to pressure on surrounding organs, bleeding or ruptures, which manifest themselves in pain reactions, sudden apathy or circulatory symptoms. In cats in particular, tumour-related disease often manifests itself in the form of unspecific general symptoms such as reduced food intake, increased withdrawal behaviour, increased sleep duration or unusual social behaviour. In everyday life, these changes are often not associated with a serious illness and therefore only lead to a late veterinary consultation.

Other important clinical indications of a possible tumour disease can be bloody or altered faeces, shortness of breath, chronic coughing, lameness without an identifiable cause, neurological abnormalities or a noticeable odour from the mouth or orifices. However, such symptoms usually only occur when the tumour has already reached a relevant size or systemic effect. In many cases, the general condition is already impaired at this point, which further complicates the prognosis.

Regular veterinary check-ups are therefore of central importance for early detection, ideally supplemented by a detailed medical history, a general clinical examination, palpation, laboratory diagnostics and, if necessary, imaging procedures. Attention to changes in the animal's behaviour or physical appearance, a willingness to clarify matters at an early stage and a trained eye for seemingly banal symptoms are crucial in order to detect tumours before they reach the final stage. Only through such a vigilant attitude can the goal of diagnosing cancer in pets in good time be achieved in order to be able to initiate the most effective therapeutic measures possible and ensure the animal's quality of life in the long term.

4.2 Organ-related manifestations and atypical courses

Behavioural changes are also an important, albeit often underestimated, diagnostic signal for the possible presence of a tumour in pets. Animals with chronic pain, a feeling of internal pressure or a general feeling of illness tend to withdraw, interact less or spend more time resting. They sleep more, show a reduced desire to play and exercise or develop increased irritability. These changes are difficult for many pet owners to categorise, as they are not specific to cancer but can also occur in other systemic or chronic diseases. Nevertheless, they are of great importance as they are often among the first signs that become noticeable in everyday behaviour. Careful veterinary clarification is therefore essential in order to identify the cause of these behavioural changes and, if necessary, to avoid overlooking an oncological disease.

In particularly sensitive cases, the symptoms also affect the central nervous system. Animals with brain tumours or other neoplasms of the central nervous system can develop neurological abnormalities. These include, for example, balance disorders, so-called ataxias, uncoordinated movements, seizures or unusual behavioural changes such as apathy, aggression or disorientation. A tilted head can also be an indication of a neurological tumour disease. Such changes require differentiated and usually complex diagnostics, in particular using imaging procedures such as magnetic resonance imaging or computer tomography, as clinical symptoms alone are often not sufficient to determine the exact cause.

Another frequently observed symptom of tumorous diseases is an increasing lack of performance or exercise intolerance. Animals that previously enjoyed exercise suddenly show a lack of interest in going for walks, refuse to play or need more rest than usual. This reduced physical resilience can also manifest itself in the form of shortness of breath, accelerated breathing or an increased need for rest. In older animals in particular, there is a risk that such changes will be misinterpreted as normal signs of age . This often leads to veterinary clarification being carried out too late, although an early diagnosis would enable a significantly better prognosis for many types of tumour. The mistake of equating age-related weakness with harmless progression can therefore have serious consequences if a treatable tumour disease is behind it.

However, in addition to the non-specific general symptoms, there are also tumour types that show very specific clinical manifestations. Mammary tumours in bitches and cats typically manifest themselves as palpable lumps along the mammary glands. These lumps can be hard or irregular, ulcerate or become inflamed and even purulent. With advanced disease, the surrounding tissue is often painful and the tumour can infiltrate into neighbouring structures. Timely surgical removal of small tumours that have not yet metastasised offers good chances of recovery in many cases.

Tumours of the oral cavity, such as malignant melanomas or squamous cell carcinomas, often manifest themselves through persistent bad breath, increased salivation, difficulty swallowing and chewing or bloody saliva. The affected animals often show one-sided food intake, salivate when eating or avoid solid food. As the oral cavity is often not thoroughly inspected during daily care, such tumours remain undetected for a long time, although they can quickly destroy the surrounding tissue due to their aggressive nature.

Bone tumours, especially osteosarcomas, on the other hand, usually cause clearly visible lameness, swelling and intense pain in the affected limbs. This pain may be intermittent at first, but increases in intensity over time and eventually barely responds to painkillers. Such lameness should always be taken seriously and not hastily equated with arthritic complaints or simple strains, especially if it increases in a short period of time or is accompanied by palpable changes to the bone.

Lymphomas, on the other hand, are often characterised by a generalised enlargement of the lymph nodes. This enlargement usually affects several lymph nodes simultaneously and in many cases is symmetrically arranged, for example in the groin area, on the neck or under the armpits.

It can be accompanied by non-specific symptoms such as loss of appetite, fever, fatigue or weight loss. As lymphomas are often systemic, internal organs such as the liver, spleen or bone marrow are also affected, which can lead to a variety of additional symptoms.

Overall, the clinical manifestations of tumour diseases in pets are extremely diverse. They range from subtle changes in behaviour to clear, localised symptoms. The key to successful diagnosis and treatment is a combination of vigilant observation, sound veterinary examination and the targeted use of modern diagnostic methods. This is the only way to ensure that the affected animals receive timely and appropriate care and enjoy the highest possible quality of life despite their illness.

4.3   Differences in symptoms between dogs and cats

The species-specific differences in clinical tumour symptoms are of great practical relevance, as they have a significant influence on early detection, diagnostic assessment and ultimately also on treatment decisions. Dogs and cats differ not only in their biology and behaviour, but also in the way they show pain, discomfort or pathological changes. This different expressive behaviour has a direct impact on veterinary diagnostics and requires a species-specific approach.

Dogs generally show clearer and often early recognisable symptoms. Clinical signs are relatively obvious in many types of tumours: lameness in bone tumours such as osteosarcoma occurs quickly, as the animals relieve the affected limbs, adopt protective postures or react to the strain by making pain sounds such as whimpering or yelping. Skin or subcutaneous tumours, which are common in mast cell tumours, for example, are discovered relatively early due to their visibility and palpability. These tumours appear as firm lumps, change in shape and size and are often associated with redness, itching or local signs of inflammation. Many dogs react sensitively to touch or pressure in the affected area, which makes diagnosis easier. Behavioural changes are also often noticeable in dogs: a decrease in the joy of movement, restlessness, increased panting or conspicuous body postures can indicate a painful tumour and lead to a veterinary consultation comparatively early on.

Cats, on the other hand, often hide illnesses for a very long time. This is not only due to their evolutionary tendency to be discreet about pain, but also to their ability to compensate for discomfort over long periods of time. Reduced appetite, increased withdrawal behaviour, altered sleeping habits or a gradual decline in physical condition are typical but very subtle signs that are easily overlooked or misinterpreted as age-related. Even in the case of internal tumours, cats often show no specific symptoms until well into the course of the disease. This late symptomatology means that tumours in cats are often only diagnosed at an advanced stage, which limits the therapeutic options and significantly worsens the prognosis. Careful observation by owners and regular check-ups are therefore particularly important in cats in order to recognise changes at an early stage.

A particularly cat-specific example is vaccine-associated fibrosarcoma. This type of tumour develops preferentially at injection sites, particularly in the neck or shoulder area, and initially appears as a slowly growing, usually painless swelling under the skin. Due to their firm consistency and slow growth, these changes are often not taken seriously or are mistaken for harmless reactions. However, the tricky thing about vaccine-associated fibrosarcoma is its aggressive biology: despite initially being harmless, these tumours tend to grow infiltratively, are often difficult to completely remove surgically and have a high risk of local recurrence. The early identification of such changes therefore requires not only a particularly trained eye, but also a sound knowledge of the typical tumour forms in cats. In veterinary practice, this has led to the development of new vaccination techniques, modified application sites and the recommendation of careful monitoring of injection sites.

In summary, it can be said that the symptoms of tumour diseases are highly species-specific. While dogs usually show clear physical or behavioural signs at an early stage, many tumour diseases in cats are initially silent or are barely noticed from the outside. This requires particularly differentiated diagnostics, adapted to the respective animal species, and a high level of attention to seemingly banal changes. Only through this differentiated approach can tumours in both species be detected in good time and treated with appropriate therapeutic measures.

4.4 Behaviour and pain as diagnostic indicators

The role of pain as a diagnostic and prognostic feature in tumour diseases in pets can hardly be overestimated. Pain is a central element of the subjective experience of illness, but animals do not have the ability to communicate it directly. It is therefore crucial to recognise subtle cues and interpret them correctly. Many animals do not show pain openly, but behave cautiously or change their behaviour in subtle ways. Typical signs can be the avoidance of certain movements, the protection of individual body regions, the sudden cessation of familiar activities or the adoption of unusual lying or sitting positions. Loss of appetite, increased licking of certain parts of the body or vocalisations when touched are also serious signs of pain, which can also be tumour-related.

Tumour pain can be triggered either by the direct infiltration of tissue, by pressure on nerves or organs or by accompanying inflammatory reactions. It is not only a central issue for the quality of life of the affected animal, but also has direct consequences for the assessment of disease dynamics and therapeutic success. An animal that is pain-free despite advanced disease and eats normally, moves around and shows social interaction is in a different prognostic starting position than an animal with severe, untreated pain. For this reason, consistent pain therapy is not only a question of animal welfare, but also an integral part of oncological care. Adequate recognition and treatment of pain not only improves well-being, but can also positively influence secondary symptoms such as inappetence, stress or immunological weakening.

Another diagnostically and prognostically relevant feature is the dynamics of tumour development. Many tumours grow over weeks or months almost asymptomatically. Well-differentiated adenocarcinomas, for example, which develop in glandular tissue, or liposarcomas, which arise from fatty tissue, often develop slowly and only cause clinical abnormalities at a late stage. Such tumours can remain undetected for a long time if they are not discovered by chance during a routine examination or only become conspicuous due to an increase in size or functional impairment. Conversely, there are highly aggressive tumour forms such as haemangiosarcoma or small cell lymphoma, which can spread within a very short time and cause a sudden deterioration in the general condition. In such cases, acute crises often occur, which are triggered by internal haemorrhaging, organ failure or systemic reactions.

The course of a tumour disease is rarely linear. Instead, vets often observe a wave-like pattern of stable phases, gradual deterioration, acute complications and occasional remissions, during which the animal temporarily appears normal again. These fluctuations require flexible, continuously adapted care and a high level of communication between pet owners and veterinary professionals. Treatment decisions must be regularly reviewed and adapted to the changing condition of the animal. Assessing when therapy is appropriate, when palliative measures should be prioritised or when the animal is suffering and its quality of life is no longer guaranteed requires a sensitive, individualised approach.

Overall, it is clear that the symptoms of cancer in pets are extremely varied and highly individualised. Some animals show no symptoms for a long time, even though a tumour is already present, while others react very early with complex, multifactorial symptoms. The challenge for veterinary practice lies in the integration of all available information: physical examination findings, behavioural observations, laboratory values, diagnostic imaging and anamnestic evidence must be assessed in the overall picture. The trick is to translate these often unspecific indications into a differentiated overall diagnostic understanding and to draw the right conclusions.

This requires not only medical expertise, but also a high degree of empathy, powers of observation and experience.

Particularly in oncology, where many decisions must be made in the context of the individual case rather than according to a rigid scheme, close cooperation with the animal owners, precise communication about treatment goals and continuous re-evaluation of the clinical picture are crucial. This is the only way to ensure that animals with tumour diseases receive care that is not only medically sound, but also ethically responsible and focused on their quality of life.

5. Diagnostic procedures in veterinary oncology

The diagnosis of cancer in pets requires a structured and methodologically diverse approach. The aim is to differentiate between benign and malignant changes, determine the type and origin of the tumour, establish its extent and possible metastasis and enable a well-founded prognosis to be made. Veterinary oncological diagnostics are based on a combination of clinical examination, imaging procedures, cytological and histopathological analyses, laboratory medical clarification and, increasingly, genetic and digital instruments. The most important procedures are described in detail below.

5.1 General veterinary examination techniques

The first and indispensable step in the oncological diagnosis of pets is a careful and systematic general clinical examination. This examination forms the basis of all further diagnostic and therapeutic decision-making and serves not only to determine the current state of health, but also to specifically search for conspicuous signs that indicate the possible presence of tumour disease. It includes a comprehensive assessment of the animal's general condition and includes checking all relevant vital parameters such as heart rate, respiratory rate, body temperature and mucous membrane colour, as changes in these areas are often an expression of systemic diseases.

Palpation of the entire body is a key part of this initial examination. The skin, subcutaneous tissue and deeper structures are carefully palpated for swelling, lumps or hardened areas of tissue. These palpation findings provide valuable information about the presence of superficial or deeper tumours. Especially in the case of skin and soft tissue tumours, which occur relatively frequently in dogs, palpation can already provide an initial suspicion. The consistency, displaceability and delimitability of a lump provide initial clues as to whether it could be a benign or possibly malignant change.

A special focus of the physical examination is on the lymph node regions. These are of central importance, as they can be enlarged or altered at an early stage in a number of oncological diseases - particularly lymphomas, metastatic carcinomas and certain systemic tumours. The palpable lymph nodes - for example under the jaw, in the armpit, in the groin area and behind the knee - are examined in terms of size, consistency, symmetry and pain. Asymmetrical changes can also provide indications of localised tumour growth or regional metastasis. The precise examination of these regions can therefore make a decisive contribution to the early detection of lymphoma or provide indications of the spread of other tumours.

In addition to the physical examination, a thorough medical history is of great importance. It not only focuses on the pet owner's subjective perception, but also provides crucial information about the course of the disease to date. Questions about the duration and development of symptoms, changes in appetite, weight or behaviour as well as physical activity and sleeping behaviour are just as important as information about previous feeding, medication, known previous illnesses or operations. The housing conditions - i.e. whether the animal lives predominantly outdoors, has contact with other animals or is exposed to particular environmental influences - can also provide information on possible exogenous risk factors. In the case of bitches, cycle behaviour should also be specifically asked about, as this plays a decisive role in assessing the risk of hormone-dependent tumours, especially mammary tumours.

5.2 Imaging procedures: X-ray, ultrasound, CT and MRI

Imaging procedures have become an integral part of modern veterinary oncology. They provide crucial information about the presence, location, size and spread of tumours, enabling precise diagnosis, well-founded treatment planning and meaningful follow-up. Their use is individually adapted depending on the problem, localisation and technical availability and in close coordination with the clinical examination and medical history.

Conventional X-ray is one of the oldest, but still extremely important imaging procedures in oncological diagnostics. It is particularly suitable for visualising bony structures and for examining the chest, especially the lungs. If pulmonary metastases are suspected - for example in primary breast tumours, osteosarcomas or haemangiosarcomas - X-rays are a fast and reliable means of visualising suspicious lesions. It also enables the visualisation of osteolyses, i.e. dissolved bone parts, as well as periosteal reactions, which may indicate a reaction of the bone to infiltrative tumour growth. X-rays are also an important diagnostic tool in emergency medicine, for example in cases of suspected tumour-related organ rupture, internal bleeding or fluid accumulation in the chest or abdominal cavity, thanks to their rapid availability and informative value.

Sonography, i.e. ultrasound examination, has established itself as indispensable, particularly in the assessment of the abdominal organs. It allows a differentiated visualisation of parenchymal organs such as the liver, spleen, kidneys, adrenal glands, urinary bladder and gastrointestinal tract. Tumours of these organs can be easily identified in terms of their structure, extent and relationship to surrounding tissues. Sonography is non-invasive, can usually be performed without anaesthesia and can be used repeatedly to monitor progress. A particular advantage is the possibility of carrying out targeted fine-needle aspirations or tissue biopsies under ultrasound guidance. This allows samples to be obtained from suspicious lesions without the need for surgical intervention. Doppler sonography can also be used to visualise the blood flow in tumours, which can provide additional information on the biological activity of the lesion.

Computed tomography (CT) offers the advantage of extremely precise, three-dimensional visualisation of even complex anatomical regions compared to X-rays and ultrasound. It is used in particular for tumours in the head area, such as the nose, oral cavity, middle ear or lower jaw, as these regions can only be assessed to a limited extent using conventional procedures. CT has also established itself as the standard for examining the spine, chest organs and internal tumours that are difficult to access. It allows the precise localisation of tumours, their differentiation from neighbouring structures and the assessment of potential infiltrations in vessels, nerves or bones. This is particularly important for surgical planning, assessing resectability and estimating the prognosis.

Magnetic resonance imaging (MRI), on the other hand, is considered the method with the best tissue resolution in the area of soft tissue. It is therefore particularly suitable for imaging the central nervous system, i.e. the brain and spinal cord, and is the method of choice for suspected brain tumours, spinal cord lesions or infiltrative sarcomas in muscle or connective tissue. Thanks to the excellent contrasts between different types of tissue, MRI enables a particularly fine differentiation between tumours and healthy tissue. This is crucial when it comes to the precise delineation of tumour margins, for example prior to neurosurgical interventions or in the assessment of complex structures in the skull or pelvic region.

Overall, diagnostic imaging is one of the cornerstones of veterinary oncology. It not only makes it possible to visualise tumours and assess their biological impact, but also to monitor the progression of a disease during treatment and to detect treatment successes or relapses at an early stage. The choice of the appropriate procedure depends on the clinical question, the organ area to be examined and the objective of the examination - be it diagnosis, therapy planning or progression assessment. In daily practice, combinations of several procedures are often necessary in order to obtain a complete picture of the disease and to be able to initiate an individually customised, effective therapy.

5.3 Cytological and histopathological methods

Cytological examination is an important part of oncological diagnostics in veterinary medicine and offers a quick, gentle way of analysing cellular changes in suspicious tissue structures. It is usually carried out as part of a fine needle aspiration, in which cell material is removed from a palpable swelling, lymph node or mass using a thin cannula. The cell material obtained is then spread on a slide, dried, stained and examined under a microscope. This method is minimally invasive, causes hardly any pain, does not require sedation in most cases and can be carried out both in general veterinary practice and in specialised clinics. Its use is particularly valuable when a rapid assessment of the nature of a change is necessary, for example in the case of sudden swellings, generalised lymph node enlargements or to check the progress of known tumours.

The morphology of the removed cells is assessed under the microscope. Important criteria here are the shape and size of the cells, the structure and expression of the nucleus, the presence of nucleoli, the uniformity or atypicality of the cell population, the arrangement of the cells in the specimen and the number and type of mitoses. High mitotic activity, an irregular nuclear structure or the presence of multinucleated cells may indicate malignant transformation. Concomitant inflammatory reactions, necrotic areas or the presence of certain cell types - such as mast cells, atypical lymphocytes or atypical epithelial cells - also allow conclusions to be drawn about the underlying pathology. Although cytology allows an initial differentiation between benign and malignant processes in many cases and provides information on the origin of the tumour, it cannot provide comprehensive information on the infiltration behaviour, the exact tissue structure or the growth limits of a tumour.

A histopathological examination is therefore necessary for a final diagnosis, an exact tumour classification, the so-called grading - i.e. the assessment of the degree of differentiation and aggressiveness - as well as for the assessment of tumour invasion into the surrounding tissue. This is based on the analysis of entire tissue sections, which are either removed surgically as part of a biopsy or under imaging control, for example using ultrasound or CT-supported procedures. The samples obtained are fixed in a standardised procedure (usually in formalin), embedded in paraffin, processed into thin sections and stained with special dyes. The most common staining method is haematoxylin-eosin staining (H&E), which shows cell nuclei and cytoplasm in high contrast and enables the tissue architecture to be assessed.

In addition, immunohistochemical techniques are increasingly being used in modern oncology, which make it possible to visualise specific cell surface markers or intracellular proteins. These methods are particularly helpful if the morphological classification is not clear or if a more precise characterisation of the tumour is required. Special antibodies can be used, for example, to identify epithelial cells (such as carcinomas), mesenchymal cells (such as sarcomas) or lymphatic cells (such as lymphomas). Molecular markers such as Ki-67 for the determination of cell proliferation or c-kit for the diagnosis of mast cell tumours can also be detected by immunohistochemistry. This additional information is not only relevant for the correct classification of the tumour, but also has direct therapeutic consequences, for example when deciding on the use of targeted therapies or the selection of suitable chemotherapy protocols.

The histopathological examination therefore forms the central decision-making basis for all further therapeutic measures. It allows an objective assessment of the prognosis, helps to select the best possible treatment option and makes it possible to monitor the course of the disease in a differentiated manner. In conjunction with the clinical, imaging and laboratory diagnostic findings, histopathology provides a comprehensive picture of the disease and is therefore an indispensable tool in modern, evidence-based veterinary oncology. The earlier and more targeted it is used, the higher the chances of successful treatment and an improved quality of life for the affected animal.

5.4 Tumour markers, genetic tests and laboratory diagnostics

Laboratory diagnostics is a key supportive tool in veterinary oncology and often provides crucial information for the assessment of tumour diseases and their systemic effects. It supplements clinical, imaging and cytological-histological diagnostics with objective, quantifiable parameters that are of great importance both for initial assessment and for monitoring during therapy or for follow-up. The aim is not only to detect changes that are directly caused by the tumour itself, but also to identify secondary disease processes that can be caused by tumour activity, the immune response or paraneoplastic syndromes.

A central element is the haematological examination, i.e. the classic blood count. Various changes associated with tumour diseases can be observed here. Anaemia - a reduction in red blood cells - occurs, for example, in the case of chronic illness, tumour bleeding or bone marrow infiltration by malignant cells. Thrombocytopenia, i.e. a lack of platelets, can be triggered by direct involvement of the bone marrow, by increased consumption as part of inflammatory reactions or by immune-mediated processes. Leukocytosis, i.e. an increased number of white blood cells, can either be an expression of a secondary infection, an inflammatory reaction to tumour tissue or, in certain cases, a sign of a haematopoietic neoplasia such as leukaemia. Atypical cells in the peripheral blood count, altered lymphocyte subtypes or the appearance of immature blood cells can also indicate involvement of the haematopoietic system.

Serum chemistry provides additional information about the organ functions and general health of the animal. The assessment of liver and kidney function is particularly important, as many tumour diseases are associated with impairment of these organs - either through direct metastasis, pressure effects or toxic concomitant processes. Elevated liver values, such as ALT, AST or alkaline phosphatase, can indicate liver involvement, while changes in urea and creatinine levels indicate impaired kidney function. These values are also crucial for the planning of drug therapies, as many chemotherapeutic agents are metabolised hepatically or renally. In addition, inflammatory markers such as C-reactive protein (CRP) or fibrinogen allow conclusions to be drawn about the extent of systemic reactions, such as tumour necrosis, infections or paraneoplastic inflammation.

Recently, special tumour markers have become increasingly important, even if their use in veterinary practice is still limited. One example is the detection of TCC antigen in urine in transitional cell carcinomas of the urinary bladder, which can represent a non-invasive diagnostic option. Such markers make it possible to confirm the suspicion of certain tumour types or to monitor the course of the disease. Molecular genetic methods are also increasingly finding their way into veterinary diagnostics. For example, so-called clonality tests based on the polymerase chain reaction (PCR) can be carried out for certain lymphomas and enable a distinction to be made between benign, reactive lymph node enlargements and malignant lymphomas.

One particularly practical advance is the ability to directly detect genetic mutations associated with certain types of tumour. In mast cell tumours, for example, the c-kit mutation is an important diagnostic and prognostic feature. It not only influences the aggressiveness of the tumour, but also allows targeted therapeutic intervention with tyrosine kinase inhibitors that act specifically on the mutated signalling pathways. Such molecular diagnostic procedures open up new possibilities for personalised veterinary medicine, in which therapy is not only symptomatic, but also targeted to the biological characteristics of the tumour.

To summarise, it can be said that laboratory diagnostics in veterinary oncology goes far beyond a supportive function. It provides essential information for diagnosis, prognosis, therapy monitoring and risk assessment and is constantly evolving with the increasing availability of molecular and genetic testing methods. Its combination with clinical and imaging findings allows a holistic assessment of the clinical picture and thus forms an indispensable basis for modern, precise and customised cancer therapy in dogs and cats.

5.5 The role of telemedicine in the diagnosis of cancer in pets

Progressive digitalisation has brought about far-reaching changes in veterinary medicine in recent years and has significantly expanded and improved oncological diagnostics in particular. Today, the targeted use of digital technologies enables significantly more efficient, networked and higher-quality diagnostics, even beyond the boundaries of individual veterinary practices or clinics. Telemedicine is playing an increasingly central role here - particularly in so-called teleoncology, i.e. digital support in the diagnosis, treatment planning and follow-up of tumour diseases in pets.

A key advantage of digital technologies is the ability to forward imaging and microscopic findings to specialised institutions in real time or within a very short space of time. X-ray images, ultrasound images, CT and MRI data sets, as well as cytological smears and histological preparations can be digitised and transmitted via secure platforms to specialised laboratories, university veterinary clinics or experienced veterinarians. This digital communication enables rapid assessment by experts who would otherwise not be available regionally. This opens up new diagnostic and therapeutic options, particularly in less specialised practices or in rural regions where complex oncological diagnostics were previously only possible to a limited extent. Receiving a well-founded second opinion within a short period of time not only improves diagnostic certainty, but also helps to build trust between the vet, pet owner and treating team.

Telemedicine also enables interdisciplinary case conferences to be held, in which various specialists - from imaging, oncology, surgery or pathology, for example - work together to develop treatment strategies. This collaborative form of case discussion contributes to a holistic, individually tailored treatment approach and guarantees comprehensive care, even for complex tumour diseases. Digital platforms also offer the possibility of documenting the course of treatment in a structured manner, integrating findings and laboratory values and analysing the course of the disease over longer periods of time. This is particularly important for chronic, slowly progressing or recurring tumour diseases.

Another forward-looking field is the use of artificial intelligence (AI) in digital diagnostics. Initial applications already enable the automated evaluation of X-ray images, the classification of cytological cell images or the analysis of histopathological sections. These processes are still in the early stages of development, but show great potential to further support veterinary diagnostics and make standardised, reproducible assessments widely accessible.

Overall, teleoncology is a promising addition to traditional oncological diagnostics. It contributes to faster, more differentiated decision-making, promotes the networking of practices and clinics and enables low-threshold access to highly specialised expertise. At a time of increasing specialisation and growing technical possibilities, it offers the potential to sustainably improve the quality of cancer diagnosis and treatment in veterinary medicine - for the benefit of the affected animals and to support the treating specialists in their everyday diagnostic and therapeutic work.

6. Classification and staging of tumours

The precise classification and exact staging of tumours in pets is an essential prerequisite for choosing an appropriate therapeutic strategy and assessing the prognosis. While the diagnosis of a tumour disease indicates that a neoplastic process is present, it is the classification that provides information about the type of tumour, the tissue from which it originated and the biological aggressiveness to be expected. The staging in turn provides information about the spread in the organism, i.e. tumour size, depth of invasion, lymph node involvement and possible metastasis. Both aspects - histological typing and clinical staging - together form the foundation of all therapeutic decision-making in veterinary oncology.

6.1 TNM system in veterinary medicine

The systematic classification of tumours into stages is a decisive step in the structured diagnosis, treatment planning and prognosis assessment of oncological diseases. In veterinary medicine, the so-called TNM system has become established, which originally comes from human medicine and has been successfully transferred to animal patients in an adapted form . This internationally recognised scheme allows a uniform description of the disease stage and thus not only facilitates interdisciplinary communication, but also the comparability of clinical studies and the derivation of standardised treatment strategies.

The acronym TNM stands for the three central diagnostic parameters: Tumour (T), Nodus (N) and Metastases (M). Each of these parameters describes a specific aspect of tumour behaviour and together contribute to the overall assessment of tumour extent and biological progression of the disease. The T-status refers to the primary tumour and describes its size and the extent of local infiltration. The scale ranges from T0 - which means that no visible or measurable primary tumour is detectable - to T1 and T2, which denote small to medium-sized tumours with no or limited invasion, to T3 and T4, which characterise large tumours with extensive infiltration of surrounding tissue or organs. This classification is not only important for the assessment of surgical resectability, but also provides information on the biological aggressiveness of the tumour.

The N-status deals with the involvement of the regional lymph nodes. Lymph nodes are often the first sites for the metastasis of tumour cells, particularly in carcinomas and some forms of sarcomas. A finding of N0 means that no involvement is detectable, while N1 and N2 represent increasing infiltration of the lymph nodes. The exact differentiation is based on the size, number and histopathological depth of invasion of the affected lymph nodes. Examination of the lymph nodes - whether by palpation, imaging or biopsy - is therefore a central component of every oncological examination and provides essential prognostic information.

Finally, the M status describes the presence or absence of distant metastases, i.e. tumour metastases in organs or tissues that are not in the immediate vicinity of the primary tumour. M0 stands for the absence of such metastases, M1 for their detection, for example in the lungs, liver, bones or brain. The detection of metastases has a direct impact on the choice and objectives of therapy - while localised tumours can often be treated curatively, metastatic disease usually requires palliative or systemic therapy concepts.

Despite its standardisation, the full application of the TNM system in veterinary practice is not always possible without restrictions. Technical limitations - such as the limited availability of high-resolution imaging or specialised laboratory diagnostics - as well as economic factors that influence diagnostic measures can make implementation difficult. Nevertheless, the TNM system provides a valuable framework for systematically recording the extent of a tumour disease and, based on this, developing a graduated, comprehensible treatment plan. It provides orientation in the assessment of the clinical course, facilitates communication with animal owners and with referring or co-treating colleagues and contributes to the structuring of oncological decision-making processes.

In addition, the use of the TNM system allows a differentiated prognosis assessment that goes beyond generalised statements. An animal with a T1N0M0 tumour generally has a much more favourable prognosis and a wider therapeutic window than a patient with a T3N2M1 stage. This differentiated assessment enables an individually tailored therapy that takes into account the biological situation of the tumour as well as the quality of life of the animal, the expectations of the owners and the feasible medical options. In this sense, the TNM system is an important building block on the way to modern, structured and patient-centred oncological care in veterinary medicine.

6.2 Grading and histology of tumours

In addition to staging using the TNM system, the grading of a tumour is an equally central parameter in oncological assessment, as it provides important information about the biological aggressiveness and expected behaviour of a tumour disease. In contrast to staging, which describes the degree of spread of a tumour in the body, grading concentrates on the microscopic properties of the tumour cells and provides information on the extent to which these cells differ from the healthy tissue of origin. Grading is carried out as part of the histopathological examination of tissue samples and, in combination with tumour classification, forms an essential basis for individual treatment planning.

The central criteria for histological grading are cell differentiation, mitotic activity, the size and shape of the cell nuclei, the ratio of cell nucleus to cytoplasm (nucleus/plasma ratio) and the preservation or loss of typical tissue architecture. Well-differentiated tumours have a cell and tissue structure that is still relatively similar to the original tissue. The cells appear organised, their nuclei are uniformly shaped and the division rate is low. Such tumours generally show slow growth and a lower potential for invasion and metastasis. They are classified as low-grade (grade I) and often have a favourable prognosis.

On the other hand, there are poorly differentiated or undifferentiated tumours in which the original tissue structure is barely recognisable. The cells are irregular, show pronounced atypia, have large or multiple cell nuclei and have high mitotic activity, which indicates rapid cell growth. These tumours are usually aggressive, infiltrate the surrounding tissue, metastasise early and often respond only to a limited extent to surgical measures. They are classified as high-grade (grade III) and usually require comprehensive, multimodal therapy, which may include chemotherapy, radiotherapy or targeted drugs in addition to surgery. Tumours with an intermediate degree of differentiation (grade II) lie between these two extremes in terms of prognosis and treatment and require careful individual assessment.

The grading therefore has a direct impact on the prognosis and therapeutic strategy. While a low-grade tumour may be considered cured by complete surgical removal, additional measures must be taken to control the spread of high-grade tumours, prevent relapses and maintain the animal's quality of life. In veterinary practice, grading is particularly important for mammary tumours, mast cell tumours, lymphomas and soft tissue sarcomas, as these tumour types occur particularly frequently and can vary greatly in their biological behaviour. Differentiated grading is essential here in order to decide on the therapeutic approach and to be able to give pet owners sound advice.

In addition, histological examination enables precise classification of the tumour according to its tissue of origin, which is of fundamental importance for understanding the disease and selecting suitable forms of therapy. Epithelial tumours, i.e. carcinomas, originate from skin, glandular or mucosal epithelia and often tend towards lymphogenous metastasis. Mesenchymal tumours or sarcomas originate from connective, muscle, bone or fatty tissue and tend to metastasise haematogenously. Haematopoietic neoplasms such as lymphomas or leukaemias affect the haematopoietic and lymphatic system and usually spread systemically. Neuroendocrine tumours, which arise from hormone-producing cells, are comparatively rare but biologically highly active and diagnostically challenging.

So-called mixed tumours, which are not so rare in animals - especially in the area of the mammary gland - also deserve special attention. These neoplasms consist of parts of different tissue types, such as epithelial and mesenchymal components, and place high demands on histological diagnostics. Their biological relevance varies, which is why precise subtyping and grading is also of great importance in these cases.

Overall, grading in conjunction with histological classification makes a decisive contribution to understanding the biological dynamics of a tumour, assessing the course of the disease and developing a targeted, evidence-based therapy. It is therefore at the heart of a modern, individualised oncological concept that is based not only on clinical symptoms but also on sound tissue and cell biology. The quality of this diagnostic assessment is decisive for therapeutic success and is a key element of any professional tumour treatment in veterinary medicine.

6.3 Relevance of staging for treatment decisions

The staging of a tumour is a central pillar in veterinary oncology decision-making and forms the basis for the individual treatment planning of each affected animal. It not only serves the medical structuring of the course of the disease, but also represents a bridge between diagnostics, therapy, prognosis and communication with the animal owners.

The systematic assessment of tumour size, lymph node involvement and metastasis allows a differentiated evaluation of which therapeutic options are realistic, what risks exist and what the aim of treatment should be.

A localised tumour in which neither involvement of the regional lymph nodes nor distant metastases can be detected may offer the chance of complete surgical removal. In such cases, treatment can be curative, i.e. aimed at complete healing. In addition to the technical possibility of complete resection, this also requires precise preoperative imaging in order to determine the actual extent and local infiltration behaviour of the tumour. If the tumour is well defined, small and limited to the original tissue, surgery alone may be sufficient in many cases to achieve a permanent remission or cure.

The situation is completely different for advanced tumours that have already grown into surrounding tissue, have metastasised to lymph nodes or have distant metastases. In these cases, curative therapy is rarely possible and the treatment approach shifts to a multimodal strategy. This includes surgical interventions to reduce the tumour mass, systemic chemotherapy to combat disseminated tumour cells, targeted molecular therapies for genetically characterised tumours and radiotherapy for local control of non-operable lesions. Such therapy combinations require differentiated planning, an interdisciplinary approach and continuous evaluation of the course of therapy.

The tumour stage also significantly influences the choice of surgical technique. While tissue-sparing surgery may be possible for small tumours with clear boundaries, infiltrative or poorly defined tumours require a more extensive resection with safety margins. The question of whether and to what extent lymph nodes should be surgically removed also depends directly on the staging. In the case of tumours with a high metastatic potential, such as mast cell tumours or malignant breast tumours, prophylactic or therapeutic lymph node removal is an important part of the overall therapy. The stage also influences the indication for further imaging procedures such as CT or MRI, particularly in the case of unclear lymph node diagnostics or suspected organ metastases.

The staging also has a direct influence on the urgency of therapeutic measures. A fast-growing, metastatic tumour requires rapid action and a clearly structured approach, while in the case of slow-growing, localised tumours with low biological activity, a controlled assessment and, if necessary, a wait-and-see strategy may be appropriate. The tumour stage therefore allows medically justified prioritisation, helps with resource planning and is indispensable for responsible decision-making.

Stage categorisation also plays a central role in discussions with pet owners. It creates transparency about the severity of the disease, enables a realistic assessment of the chances of success and promotes the joint development of a therapeutic goal. Whether a cure is sought, the longest possible tumour-free interval is achieved or only the quality of life is maintained depends crucially on how advanced the disease is at the time of diagnosis. The classification of the tumour in a comprehensible scheme provides structure, creates orientation and is an essential basis for informed consent to therapeutic measures.

Last but not least, the tumour stage is also a decisive prognostic factor. Numerous studies have shown that it is the single strongest predictor of long-term survival and the expected quality of life of the affected animal. The earlier a tumour is detected and classified, the higher the chances of successful treatment. Precise staging, which sensibly integrates all available diagnostic methods, enables an individualised, evidence-based treatment strategy and is therefore a central instrument of modern veterinary medicine. It not only contributes to medical quality assurance, but also promotes ethically responsible decision-making processes - for the benefit of the animal and in respectful dialogue with the people caring for it.

6.4 Prognosis estimation and individual progression expectation

The prognosis for tumour diseases in pets is the result of a complex interplay of numerous medical, biological and individual factors, which together determine the course, life expectancy, quality of life and therapeutic prospects. It is not just a matter of estimating the survival time, but rather a comprehensive view of the clinical picture that takes into account both medical-objective criteria and the subjective life situation of the animal and the possibilities of its carers.

The exact type of tumour is of central importance for the prognosis. Each neoplasm follows its own biological pattern, which is determined by the speed of growth, invasion behaviour, tendency to metastasise and response to therapy. For example, well-differentiated breast tumours or subcutaneous lipomas often have an excellent prognosis if completely removed, whereas aggressive forms such as haemangiosarcomas, osteosarcomas or high-grade lymphomas often have a limited life expectancy even with intensive therapy. Histological grading, which provides information on the extent to which the tumour cells differ from the healthy original tissue, is closely linked to this. Low grading indicates slower tumour progression, while high grading indicates an aggressive biology and an increased risk of relapse or metastasis.

The clinical stage of the disease at the time of diagnosis is one of the most important individual predictors of prognosis. A localised tumour detected at an early stage can often be treated curatively, while advanced tumours with systemic spread can in many cases only be controlled palliatively. The more precisely the extent of the tumour is detected using imaging techniques and lymph node examinations, the more precisely the prognosis can be formulated and the therapeutic approach planned. The biological aggressiveness of the tumour also plays a role here, which is determined not only by grading, but also by molecular characteristics such as certain mutations, proliferation markers or the response to immunological control mechanisms.

The genetic make-up of tumours is increasingly the subject of intensive research. Mutations in certain genes - such as c-kit in mast cell tumours - not only influence the biological behaviour of the tumour, but also open up therapeutic options with targeted drugs. The animal's immune response, i.e. its ability to recognise and eliminate tumour cells, also plays a significant role, particularly in the application of immunological or immunomodulatory therapies.

Patient-related factors also have a significant influence on the prognosis. Age, general state of health, presence of concomitant diseases, resilience and ability to recover influence not only the suitability for treatment, but also the quality of life during and after treatment. A young, immunocompetent dog with no previous illnesses will have a different prognosis under the same tumour conditions than a geriatric patient with cardiac or metabolic comorbidity.

Another key influencing factor is the availability of effective therapeutic measures. Whether surgical removal is possible, whether chemotherapy is available, whether radiotherapy or targeted medication can be used depends not only on the type of tumour, but also on the organisational and financial framework conditions. Equally important is the response of the tumour to the therapy that has been initiated, which should be checked regularly during follow-up using clinical, laboratory diagnostic and imaging procedures. Tumours that shrink or stabilise under therapy have a much more favourable prognosis than those that are resistant or progressive.

The prognosis assessment serves not only to soberly estimate life expectancy, but also to assess the expected quality of life, the risk of relapse, the burden of treatment and the prospect of symptom-free or at least symptom-free intervals. Modern prognosis models attempt to structure this complex wealth of factors using multivariate analyses and decision trees so that a more individualised and differentiated prognosis is possible. They integrate medical data with ethical, emotional and practical aspects and thus enable animal-centred, responsible decision-making.

It is crucial for the attending veterinarian to communicate these prognostic assessments openly, empathetically and professionally with the animal owners at . The prognosis must not be understood as a rigid number or as a mere medical value, but must be embedded in the context of the individual case. The aim should always be to jointly develop a treatment plan that respects both the welfare of the animal and the possibilities, wishes and limitations of the people caring for it.

The combination of scientifically sound staging, differentiated prognosis assessment and empathetic support thus forms the basis of all responsible veterinary oncology. It ensures that treatment decisions are not only medically justified, but also humanly comprehensible and ethically justifiable - and thus fulfil the requirements of modern, holistic veterinary medicine.

7. Therapeutic approaches and healing methods

The treatment of cancer in pets is a dynamic, interdisciplinary field that has developed considerably in recent decades. Whereas in the past the only choice was often between euthanasia or surgical removal, modern veterinary oncology now offers a wide range of therapeutic options, including surgical, drug, radiotherapeutic, immunological, cell-based and palliative medical procedures. The aim of these treatments is not only to prolong life, but also - and increasingly in the foreground - to maintain or restore the quality of life of the diseased animal. The decision for a particular form of therapy depends on the type of tumour, the stage of the disease, the general condition of the animal, the prognostic assessment and the individual options and wishes of the pet owner.

7.1 Surgical forms of therapy and their limitations

Surgical removal of a tumour is still one of the most effective and most frequently used treatment options in veterinary oncology, especially for localised tumours without signs of metastasis. If the general condition of the animal is stable, the anatomical position of the tumour allows surgical access and complete removal with a sufficient safety margin appears possible, the curative intention is paramount. The aim of the operation in such cases is the complete excision of all tumour cells, which can potentially lead to a complete cure. This approach is particularly relevant for tumours such as soft tissue sarcomas, mast cell tumours or breast tumours, as these can often be completely resected if diagnosed at an early stage and surgical removal can provide an excellent prognosis.

However, preoperative planning requires in-depth knowledge of the specific tumour behaviour, particularly with regard to its growth and invasion pattern. Tumours differ considerably in how they expand into the surrounding tissue, whether they are clearly demarcated or grow in a diffusely infiltrating manner and whether they form microscopic satellite foci. These biological characteristics largely determine the surgical strategy and the necessary safety margin required to achieve a tumour-free resection area. Precise diagnostic imaging - such as sonography, CT or MRI - is therefore essential in order to fully assess the extent of the tumour and plan the surgical steps precisely.

Despite all the advances in surgical technology, surgical tumour removal reaches its limits in certain tumour locations or advanced stages of the disease. Tumours that are located in anatomically difficult-to-access regions such as the brain, within the rib cage, in the pelvic cavity or in the area of the spine can often only be resected to a limited extent. The high risk of surgical complications, such as vascular injuries, damage to functionally important nerves or organs, limits the radical nature of the procedure. Infiltrating tumours that affect several types of tissue or organs at the same time, or tumours that are already present in the form of multiple foci, cannot be completely removed in many cases.

In such situations, the concept of debulking surgery is often used. The tumour is not reduced completely, but only in its mass, in order to alleviate the clinical symptoms, improve the quality of life or increase the effectiveness of subsequent forms of therapy such as chemotherapy or radiotherapy. Debulking operations can be particularly useful in animals with a heavy tumour burden, painful or obstructive tumours or to control local progression, even if they do not have a curative effect. They often serve as part of a multimodal therapy concept and require close coordination with other specialist disciplines.

Tumour surgery always requires careful pre-operative preparation, a high level of surgical expertise and close post-operative care. Factors such as anaesthetic capability, blood coagulation, immunological stability and wound healing potential must be clarified in advance. During the procedure, a precise technique is required to minimise bleeding, preserve tissue and achieve an exact tumour resection with adequate margins. Intraoperative assessment of tumour margins - for example by rapid staining - can help to verify the completeness of the removal.

Intensive follow-up care is necessary after the operation in order to recognise and treat possible complications at an early stage. Wound healing disorders, serous fluid accumulation, secondary bleeding or infections can not only impair the animal's well-being, but also worsen the oncological prognosis. The question of whether the tumour margins are assessed as "clean" - i.e. tumour-free - in the histopathological findings is particularly critical. If tumour cells are detectable at the resection margin, the risk of local recurrence increases significantly, which may necessitate further surgery or adjuvant therapy.

In many cases, surgical therapy is therefore combined with other forms of treatment to reduce the risk of recurrence or to combat systemic tumour cells. Postoperative chemotherapy may be indicated, for example, if a tumour has a high metastatic potential or if lymph nodes have already been affected. Radiotherapy of the surgical site can also be useful, particularly for tumours with narrow or not completely clean resection margins or tumours that show a high tendency to relapse.

Overall, surgical therapy is a central element of veterinary oncological care, which in many cases offers the best chance of cure or long-term control. However, its success depends on a variety of factors: the tumour biology, the anatomical location, the general condition of the animal, surgical experience and adequate post-operative care. As part of a holistic therapy concept, it must always be individually planned, carefully carried out and closely monitored - for the benefit of the animal and in awareness of the possibilities and limitations that this form of therapy entails.

7.2 Radiotherapy in small animal oncology

Radiotherapy is a highly specialised, technically sophisticated and extremely effective treatment option in veterinary oncology, which is used in particular in cases where surgical measures are not possible, insufficient or associated with too great a risk. It is based on the principle of irreversibly damaging tumour cells through the targeted application of ionising radiation by damaging their DNA to such an extent that the cells can no longer divide and ultimately die. Great importance is attached to protecting the surrounding healthy tissue, which is made possible by precise planning, computer-aided simulations and modern radiation technologies such as linear accelerators.

These linear accelerators generate high-energy photon radiation that can be focused precisely on the affected tumour area. Computer-aided radiation planning allows the dose distribution in the animal's body to be controlled so that the maximum dose reaches the tumour tissue, while neighbouring organs are spared as far as possible. Radiotherapy is usually carried out in several fractions - i.e. over a series of sessions - which not only increases effectiveness but also reduces the risk of side effects. This approach is based on the principle that tumour cells recover less well from radiation damage than healthy cells, which are given time to regenerate between fractions.

Radiotherapy is particularly indicated for tumours that cannot be surgically removed or can only be removed with unacceptable functional losses. These include tumours in the head and neck area - such as nasal, ear or laryngeal tumours -, intracranial or intraspinal tumours and tumours in the oral cavity, orbit or paranasal sinuses. The spread of residual tumours after incomplete surgical removal can also be limited or even completely controlled by postoperative radiotherapy. Furthermore, radiotherapy is playing an increasingly important role in palliative care, particularly in the case of painful bone metastases or tumours that exert pressure on neighbouring structures due to their size, causing pain, respiratory distress or neurological deficits. In these cases, radiotherapy can improve quality of life, alleviate symptoms and give the animal a much more comfortable remaining life.

However, radiation treatment requires a specialised setting. It is technically complex, requires precise pre-planning using CT or MRI imaging, elaborate positioning of the animal during radiotherapy and usually repeated sedation or anaesthesia to ensure exact positioning. As animals do not understand the need to remain still, each session usually has to be carried out under short anaesthesia. The entire duration of treatment often extends over several weeks, which can be a great burden both organisationally and also emotionally and financially.

Although radiotherapy is very effective when indicated, it is not free of side effects. The most common acute reactions include skin irritation, inflammation of the mucous membranes, local swelling or temporary fatigue. These symptoms usually occur within the first few weeks of starting treatment and are generally reversible. In the long term, however, late effects such as fibrosis, permanent pigment changes or restrictions in the function of irradiated organs can also occur. These risks depend on the dose, the location of the tumour and the sensitivity of the affected tissue. A careful risk-benefit assessment and close supervision by experienced radiotherapists are therefore essential.

Last but not least, radiotherapy also represents a considerable economic investment. The high purchase and operating costs of the equipment, the personnel requirements and the complex planning mean that this form of treatment is generally only offered in specialised oncology centres. For pet owners, this is not only a financial challenge, but also a logistical one, especially if long journeys are required.

This makes close cooperation between the referring vet, the radiotherapy team and the pet owners all the more important. Open communication about the goals, the procedure, the possible side effects and the prognosis of the therapy is the basis for a responsible decision. The welfare of the animal should always take centre stage - with the aim of not only prolonging life, but above all maintaining or restoring quality of life. Radiotherapy can make a decisive contribution in this context - provided that it is carefully planned, competently carried out and individually tailored to the respective patient.

7.3 Chemotherapy: protocols, active substances and side effects

In veterinary oncology, chemotherapy is a central instrument for the treatment of systemic tumour diseases and is an essential therapeutic option, particularly for disseminated, inoperable or metastatic neoplasia. Its effectiveness is based on the targeted damage to tumour cells by cytotoxic substances that interfere with cell division and thus inhibit tumour growth or lead to cell death. The aim is to destroy tumour cells as selectively as possible or to permanently interrupt their proliferation without causing excessive damage to healthy tissue. In veterinary practice, the balance between therapeutic effectiveness and good tolerability is paramount.

Chemotherapy is used particularly frequently for haematopoietic tumours such as lymphomas and leukaemias, as these diseases are typically systemic and surgical treatment is either not possible or not appropriate. Chemotherapy is also a relevant treatment option for metastasised carcinomas in which distant metastases have been detected in the lungs, liver, bones or other organs. It can also be used as an adjuvant measure following surgical removal of the tumour to eliminate any remaining microscopic tumour cells and reduce the risk of recurrence.

In veterinary medicine, chemotherapy is used in significantly adjusted dosages compared to human medicine. The main objective is not maximum cytotoxic effect, but effective control of the tumour disease with the least possible stress on the animal. The dosages and intervals are individually adapted to the respective animal species, body weight, type of tumour, stage of disease, response to therapy and general condition of the patient. This allows a good quality of life to be maintained during treatment in many cases.

The most commonly used chemotherapeutic agents include vincristine, a mitosis inhibitor from the vinca alkaloid group, doxorubicin, an anthracycline with a broad spectrum of activity, cyclophosphamide, an alkylating cytostatic agent, and carboplatin, a platinum-containing DNA-damaging agent. For certain indications, L-asparaginase is also used, an enzyme that is particularly effective in lymphomas by removing vital amino acids from the tumour cells. The selection of substances and the structure of the treatment are based on standardised protocols that are regularly adapted to the course of therapy. A well-known example is the CHOP protocol for malignant lymphomas, which involves a combination of cyclophosphamide, hydroxydaunorubicin (doxorubicin), vincristine and prednisone and has proven effective in numerous studies.

In contrast to human medicine, serious side effects occur less frequently in animals, which is due to the more conservative dosage, the better general condition of many animal patients and the more targeted application. Nevertheless, side effects cannot be ruled out and must be integrated into the overall therapeutic concept. The most common adverse effects include gastrointestinal symptoms such as nausea, vomiting or diarrhoea, which can be caused by damage to rapidly proliferating mucosal cells. Temporary apathy, refusal to eat or an increased need to rest may also occur. Hair loss is much rarer in animals than in humans, but can occur in certain breeds - especially those with continuous hair growth. Bone marrow depression with reduced production of white blood cells, red blood cells and platelets is a potentially serious side effect and requires close monitoring of blood counts during treatment. Liver or kidney dysfunctions are also possible and must be taken into account, particularly with prolonged or high-dose therapy.

Chemotherapy is monitored by regular clinical examinations, blood count checks and, if necessary, laboratory analyses of liver and kidney values. This is the only way to ensure early detection and control of side effects. The decision for or against chemotherapy must always be made on an individual basis and weighed up responsibly in dialogue with the animal owners.

A key aspect of this is the acceptance of the therapy by the pet owner, as emotional, organisational and financial factors also play a significant role alongside medical considerations. Regular visits to a specialised clinic, the need for frequent blood tests and injections as well as the psychological burden of being confronted with a serious diagnosis can be challenging. Open, transparent communication about the opportunities, limitations and expected side effects of treatment is therefore essential in order to jointly develop a treatment concept that is not only medically sensible, but also practically feasible and ethically acceptable.

Chemotherapy is therefore a highly effective treatment option that is used responsibly, individually adapted and under continuous monitoring in modern veterinary medicine. Its aim is not only to prolong survival, but above all to maintain the best possible quality of life for the diseased animal. In combination with other forms of therapy and taking into account all accompanying factors, it offers a valuable opportunity to give many animal cancer patients a life worth living.

7.4 Immunotherapy, targeted therapy and personalised approaches

A comparatively young but rapidly growing field within veterinary oncology is immune and molecularly targeted therapy, which has the potential to fundamentally change the treatment of tumour diseases in pets. At the heart of these approaches is the desire to no longer exclusively destroy the tumour cells themselves, but to use the biological properties of the tumour in a targeted manner and to involve the body's own immune system in the fight or to direct it pharmacologically. This development reflects an increasing convergence with the principles of personalised medicine, as already established in human oncology, and marks a paradigm shift towards individualised, biologically based therapy strategies.

The aim of immunotherapy is to modulate the immune system so that it recognises and effectively combats tumour cells without affecting healthy tissue. Various strategies are used, such as the activation of cellular immune responses, the use of tumour-specific vaccines or the application of monoclonal antibodies. In veterinary medicine, this form of therapy has so far been particularly advanced in the treatment of certain melanomas. For example, a vaccine based on tyrosinase-containing antigens has already been authorised for canine malignant oral melanomas. It is designed to stimulate the animal's immune system to act specifically against tumour cells that express this enzyme, which is otherwise rarely found in healthy tissue. Experience to date with such immunotherapies is promising, even if their use has so far been limited to selected indications and specialised centres.

Another highly relevant concept is targeted molecular therapy. It is based on the pharmacological inhibition of certain signalling pathways that are permanently activated in tumour cells due to mutations or epigenetic changes. A prominent example is the use of tyrosine kinase inhibitors such as toceranib, a drug that is used in particular for mast cell tumours with a proven c-kit mutation. This mutation leads to permanent activation of a growth receptor on the cell surface, which triggers uncontrolled cell growth. Toceranib specifically blocks this signal transmission, which can significantly slow down or even halt tumour growth. As these drugs act specifically on tumour-associated mechanisms, they are generally better tolerated and have fewer systemic side effects than conventional chemotherapeutic agents.

However, this form of targeted therapy requires prior molecular biological characterisation of the tumour, which can currently only be carried out in specialised laboratories. Molecular markers, gene mutations and expression profiles must be identified and interpreted in order to decide whether a targeted therapy makes sense at all. This approach marks the transition to personalised oncology, i.e. a treatment strategy that is no longer based solely on histological diagnoses, but on the individual biological signature of a tumour.

Even though this form of medicine is still in its infancy in veterinary oncology, new, forward-looking perspectives are opening up here. Advances in molecular diagnostic methods - such as next-generation sequencing or expression analyses - are making it possible to create tumour profiles in animals that enable differentiated, tailored therapies. This development not only opens up new therapeutic possibilities, but also enables an in-depth scientific examination of the tumour biology of various animal species.

At the same time, it should be emphasised that these procedures are currently still associated with considerable costs and are generally only available at university or highly specialised institutions. The integration of these therapies into everyday clinical practice will therefore only take place gradually, depending on technical availability, financial resources and the progress of research. Nevertheless, the direction is clear: veterinary oncology is increasingly moving in the direction of precise, individualised medicine, which no longer reacts only to general tumour categories, but places the genetic, molecular and immunological individuality of the tumour at the centre of treatment.

In the long term, this approach not only offers the opportunity to significantly improve the effectiveness of tumour treatment, but also to minimise side effects and significantly improve the quality of life of the animals. Immune and targeted therapy thus marks a milestone in the development of modern, responsible and future-orientated veterinary oncology.

7.5 Stem cell-based therapies and regenerative medicine

The use of stem cells in veterinary oncology represents a highly innovative and promising field of research that pursues two fundamentally different therapeutic objectives: On the one hand, stem cells are intended to contribute to the regeneration and support of the body's own repair processes after stressful oncological treatments such as chemotherapy or radiotherapy. On the other hand, research is being conducted into their direct anti-tumour or immunomodulatory effect in order to use them specifically to combat tumours. While the former application is already closer to clinical realisation, the direct tumour-inhibiting approaches are still largely at the experimental stage.

A key field of application is regenerative stem cell therapy following intensive cancer treatment. Chemotherapy and radiotherapy - despite their targeted effect against tumour cells - often also cause considerable damage to healthy tissue, particularly in highly proliferative organs such as the bone marrow, the mucous membrane of the digestive tract or the skin. In these cases, mesenchymal stem cells obtained from adipose tissue, bone marrow or umbilical cord blood can potentially contribute to regeneration by having an anti-inflammatory effect, stimulating cell division in damaged tissue and promoting tissue healing through the release of growth factors. Initial veterinary studies - for example in dogs with radiation-induced tissue damage - show positive effects on wound healing, anti-inflammation and structural regeneration, although the data is still limited and systematic long-term studies are lacking.

A second, much more experimental goal is the development of stem cell-based immunotherapies that specifically target the anti-tumour immune response. The aim here is to manipulate stem cells or stem cell-like cells - such as dendritic cells or tumour-specific T cells - in such a way that they become specifically active against tumour cells. Dendritic cells, for example, are professional antigen-presenting cells that can recognise and process tumour antigens and present them to the immune system. In studies, attempts are being made to load these cells ex vivo with tumour antigens and then administer them to the animal in order to trigger a targeted immune response against the tumour. The activation of tumour-specific cytotoxic T cells is also being investigated in this context. However, there is currently a lack of sufficiently controlled clinical studies that allow a reliable statement to be made about the effectiveness, safety and reproducibility of these procedures in veterinary medicine.

Despite the current limitations in clinical applicability, the future potential of stem cell-based therapies is enormous. They offer the possibility of developing personalised, biologically tailored treatment concepts that go beyond purely destructive tumour control and incorporate regenerative and immunological mechanisms. Particularly in the context of combined therapies - for example in conjunction with chemotherapy, immunotherapy or molecularly targeted drugs - stem cells could make a significant contribution by improving therapy tolerability, reducing side effects and possibly also strengthening tumour defence in the long term.

In the long term, the genetic modification of stem cells could also help to increase their targeting and effectiveness. In human medical research, for example, work is being carried out on CAR T cells, in which T cells are genetically modified in such a way that they recognise and attack tumour antigens particularly effectively. The transfer of such concepts to veterinary medicine is conceivable, but requires considerable technological progress and careful risk assessments.

Overall, it is clear that stem cell-based approaches - whether regenerative, immunomodulatory or directly antitumour - represent an important future field in oncology. In veterinary practice, we are still at the beginning, but ongoing research and increasing interdisciplinary cooperation between veterinary medicine, cell biology and immunology suggest that stem cells will become increasingly important as a complementary element in individualised therapy concepts in the future. Their potential lies not only in their therapeutic efficacy, but also in the possibility of further developing veterinary oncology into a more holistic, biologically based speciality.

7.6 Alternative medical methods and their scientific evaluation

The use of complementary and alternative medical procedures is also increasing in the field of animal oncology. These include phytotherapy, homeopathy, acupuncture, orthomolecular medicine, magnetic field therapy and various dietary measures. Many pet owners are looking for complementary forms of treatment, especially when conventional medical options are limited or associated with side effects.

However, the scientific evidence for the effectiveness of such procedures is often insufficient or contradictory. Individual plant substances such as artemisinin, curcumin or certain mushroom extracts show tumour-inhibiting properties in vitro, but their clinical relevance in animals has not yet been convincingly proven. The veterinary recommendation of alternative methods should therefore always be based on scientific evidence, taking into account possible interactions and as part of an integrative treatment concept.

7.7 Palliative medical measures for non-curative cases

If a cure is not possible, palliative care takes centre stage. The aim of palliative care for animals is to alleviate pain, reduce anxiety, control breathlessness, nausea or other distressing symptoms and enable the animal to enjoy the highest possible quality of life until the end of its life. Pain management, appetite stimulation, fluid administration, symptom-orientated care and stable emotional support for the owner are among the key measures.

Palliative care can be provided on an outpatient basis, in specialised facilities or at home. An open discussion about the course of the disease, possible complications, euthanasia decisions and the dying process is necessary in order to avoid unnecessary suffering and to accompany the animal and owner with dignity.

8. Quality of life, care and ethical considerations

The treatment of cancer in pets is not exclusively a medical-technical task, but also always a deeply emotional and ethical endeavour. Maintaining or restoring quality of life is at the centre of every oncological therapy, especially when curative treatment is no longer possible. The welfare of the animal must always be harmonised with the subjective assessment of the animal owner, the medical possibilities and the economic and psychological framework conditions. The question of the right balance between prolonging life and quality of life, between therapy and avoiding suffering, is one of the greatest challenges in veterinary oncology.

8.1 Quality of life assessment from a veterinary point of view

Assessing the quality of life of an animal with cancer is a particularly sensitive and complex process that involves not only medical, but also ethical, emotional and communicative components. In veterinary oncology, this assessment is of central importance, as it is directly linked to the question of whether therapy should be started, continued or possibly ended. Unlike in human medicine, where patients can describe and reflect on their quality of life in their own words, the veterinary assessment must be based on careful observation by the veterinarian and on the perception and assessment by the animal's carer.

Quality of life cannot be reduced to individual physical parameters, but requires an integrative consideration of physiological as well as psychological and social aspects. The key physical indicators include freedom from pain, mobility, normal eating behaviour, undisturbed defecation and urination, normal breathing, a well-groomed appearance and the absence of stressful symptoms such as vomiting, diarrhoea or chronic fatigue. At the same time, however, it is also important to consider how the animal perceives its environment, whether it actively participates in social life, shows interest in interactions, develops play behaviour or voluntarily enters familiar situations. The ability to move independently, to eat and to regulate resting and waking phases are also an expression of a stable physical and mental balance.

The challenge is to systematise these diverse impressions and translate them into a clinically usable form without ignoring the individual character, medical history or social behaviour of the animal in question. Structured rating scales have proven to be a helpful guide here. One frequently used method is the so-called "HHHHHHMM" scale, which focuses on seven core areas: Pain ("Hurt"), hunger, hydration ("Hydration"), hygiene (cleanliness and grooming), happiness ("Happiness"), mobility and the balance between good and bad days ("More good days than bad"). This scale is intended to enable owners and the treatment team to engage in structured reflection and help to translate subjective impressions into a comprehensible decision matrix.

However, despite its practical value, such a scale should never be used as the sole basis for decision-making. It is an aid, not a substitute for veterinary experience, empathy and clinical expertise. This is because every animal reacts differently to illness, pain or therapy. Some animals withdraw when suffering, others show hardly any noticeable behaviour even though they are in considerable pain. Individual factors such as temperament, living environment, attachment to attachment figures and previous illnesses also play a major role. The owner's subjective perception - for example through changes in behaviour, vocalisation or body language - is therefore just as valuable a source of information as the objective clinical examination.

A particularly important aspect of quality of life is the tolerability of the therapy. A medically effective measure loses its value if it is accompanied by significant side effects that place excessive strain on the animal. Chemotherapy that slows tumour growth but leads to chronic loss of appetite, weakness or gastrointestinal disorders can impair the animal's well-being to such an extent that it is no longer justifiable to continue. Continuous re-evaluation of the quality of life is therefore essential - especially in the course of longer-term treatments. Regular check-ups, discussions with the pet owners and targeted observation of the animal's behaviour are necessary in order to identify changes at an early stage and adapt therapeutic measures accordingly.

The overriding aim of any responsible veterinary cancer treatment is not just to prolong life, but to maintain or restore the best possible quality of life. In practice, this means consistently avoiding pain, treating side effects at an early stage and always keeping an eye on whether the animal still enjoys life, feels well and can organise its everyday life independently. In this area of conflict between medical possibilities, ethical responsibility and emotional attachment, the quality of life assessment is an indispensable compass - for the veterinarians treating animals as well as for the people who accompany their pets. It forms the basis for a therapy that is not only clinically appropriate, but also animal-friendly, empathetic and humanely responsible.

8.2 Communication between veterinarian, animal owner and, if applicable, psychologist

Open, respectful and empathetic communication is a basic prerequisite for the success of any oncological therapy. The vet must be able to explain medically complex issues in an understandable way, convey realistic expectations and take the pet owner's emotional reactions seriously. At the same time, it is necessary to leave room for questions, doubts and personal wishes. The discussion about the diagnosis of cancer, the possible treatment options and the prognosis should always take place in a calm and undisturbed atmosphere.

In difficult decision-making situations, it can also be useful to involve external specialists, such as psychologists specialising in animal grief counselling or palliative care specialists. Many pet owners experience their pet's cancer diagnosis as traumatic, feeling guilty or overwhelmed. Veterinary care must recognise this emotional context and must not be reduced solely to communicating facts.

Psychosocial support becomes particularly important in the end-of-life phase. The moment when therapeutic measures are postponed in favour of palliative medical care or euthanasia requires a particularly high degree of communicative sensitivity. Empathetic conversations can help to reduce feelings of guilt, promote rational decision-making and strengthen trust between vet and owner.

8.3 Ethical aspects of treatment decisions

The question of which treatment is appropriate in which situation cannot be decided solely on the basis of medical parameters. Ethical considerations must be taken into account as well as the needs of the animal and the limits of the owner. Various ethical principles are in conflict here: respect for life, the duty to avoid suffering, human responsibility for the animal and the limits of medical feasibility.

The central ethical question is: What benefits the animal? Or - in a negative sense - what is reasonable? A therapy that subjects the animal to weeks of pain, fear or considerable restrictions without any realistic prospect of a cure or relevant prolongation of life can be ethically problematic, even if it is technically feasible. In such cases, the veterinarian must have the courage to suggest that the animal should forgo therapy or be euthanised as a possible option - without pressure, but with clarity and professional authority.

The resources of the pet owner also play a role in the ethical consideration. Not every owner is in a position to finance costly treatments, organise transport and care or bear the emotional pressure over a long period of time. The ethical stance in veterinary oncology should therefore not be geared towards maximum technical care, but towards a responsible balance between medical feasibility and individual welfare.

8.4 Hospice care and end-of-life care for animals

When the time has come when a cure is ruled out and palliative care is indicated, the phase of end-of-life care begins. The aim is to enable the animal to live a dignified, pain-free and anxiety-free life until the last moment. Veterinary hospice care includes pain therapy, symptomatic treatment, psychological support for owners and organisational and medical preparation for the farewell.

During this phase, many pet owners would like their pets to be cared for at home, where they are in familiar surroundings. Home visits, mobile pain therapy and the option of euthanasia in the pet's own home are key components of animal-friendly hospice care. At the same time, information about typical dying processes, possible complications and the signs of approaching death is essential in order to avoid uncertainty and excessive demands.

The decision to euthanise should never be taken lightly, but should be made clearly, thoughtfully and on the basis of medical and ethical considerations. It is an act of compassion and an expression of responsible care when all other options have been exhausted. The veterinarian has a dual role here: he is both a medical expert and an ethical counsellor. In both functions, he bears a great responsibility for the animal and for the owner, who must accompany a painful but necessary step.

9. Prevention and health care

The prevention of cancer in pets is becoming increasingly important in view of the rising number of cases and increasing diagnostic sensitivity. While not all types of tumours can be prevented by preventive measures, it is certainly possible to significantly reduce the risk of many diseases through targeted prevention, early detection and a healthy lifestyle. In this context, prevention not only means preventing the development of tumours, but also the early identification of risk constellations, timely therapeutic intervention and the active involvement of the animal owner in maintaining animal health.

9.1 Vaccinations, castration and preventive examinations

A central component of veterinary tumour prevention is the consistent use of evidence-based prophylactic measures to reduce the risk of tumour development or enable early detection. Both medical-technical interventions such as vaccinations and castrations and organisational structures such as regular check-ups play a decisive role here. The aim of these measures is to reduce the proportion of avoidable cancers, to shift diagnosis to the earliest possible stage of the disease and to ensure the long-term quality of life of the animals through targeted health monitoring.

The vaccination strategy deserves particular attention in the context of tumour prevention, especially with regard to the vaccine-associated fibrosarcomas documented in cats. These malignant tumours develop in rare cases at the injection sites, particularly in the neck area or between the shoulder blades, and are suspected to be caused by the local reaction to certain adjuvants in vaccines. Although the absolute frequency of these tumours is low, their occurrence has nevertheless had far-reaching consequences for vaccine management. Today, vaccines with a reduced adjuvant concentration are preferred in order to minimise the local irritation potential. In addition, the practice of administering vaccines deeply subcutaneously or as distally as possible - for example in the distal area of limbs or the lateral abdominal area - has become established. If a tumour does subsequently develop, complete surgical removal at these sites is possible with significantly less risk and functional loss. Careful documentation of the vaccine, the injection site and the date of administration is not only necessary from a liability perspective , but also enables close monitoring of potential vaccination reactions.

Another highly effective approach to tumour prevention is prophylactic castration, which can have a preventative effect, particularly in the case of hormone-dependent tumours. In bitches, the risk of developing mammary tumours can be significantly reduced by spaying before the first or second heat at the latest - the earlier the procedure is performed, the more pronounced the preventive effect. Neutering has also been shown to significantly reduce the incidence of testicular tumours and perianal adenomas in male dogs. In cats, early castration not only prevents unwanted reproduction, but also prevents diseases of the uterus and hormone-related tumours. It can also reduce the occurrence of certain behavioural disorders associated with sex hormones. However, the decision to neuter should always be made taking into account the individual health status, living conditions, genetic disposition and breed background. Particularly in the case of animals that are predisposed to certain diseases or were intended as breeding animals, the benefits and possible risks must be carefully weighed up.

Another elementary pillar of cancer prevention is the regular performance of veterinary screening examinations. These are not only used for general health monitoring, but are also an indispensable tool for the early detection of tumour diseases that have not yet become clinically apparent. Older animals in particular, in which the risk of neoplasia increases significantly, should undergo a comprehensive clinical examination at least once a year. In addition to a thorough physical examination, this also includes laboratory analyses, such as blood tests to assess organ function, haematological parameters to detect systemic changes and urine analyses for the early detection of urological diseases. Depending on the findings or risk profile of the animal, imaging procedures such as X-rays, sonography or - if certain types of tumours are suspected - further diagnostics such as CT or MRI may also be indicated.

Regular screening not only enables early diagnosis, but also increases the probability that a detected tumour is still in a treatable, localised stage. This significantly improves the therapeutic options, the animal's quality of life and the prognosis. Structured preventive care also makes it possible to inform pet owners at an early stage about preventive measures, changes in behaviour or clinical abnormalities and to raise awareness of the importance of regular health monitoring.

9.2 Diet, exercise and avoidance of risk factors

A healthy lifestyle is also playing an increasingly important role in the prevention of tumour diseases in veterinary medicine. While the concept of preventive health management has long been established in humans, it is also becoming increasingly important in the care of pets, as many influencing factors that are associated with an increased risk of cancer in humans are also transferable to animals. The holistic view of nutrition, exercise, environmental conditions and behaviour makes it possible to reduce the risk of certain cancers in dogs and cats in a targeted manner and at the same time promote general well-being and quality of life throughout their entire lifespan.

Nutrition is a central component of this preventive lifestyle. Even though the scientific data in veterinary medicine is still incomplete and large-scale, controlled studies on the direct correlation between certain feed components and the development of tumours are still lacking, there are numerous indications of a potential link. In particular, the use of synthetic preservatives, artificial colourings or low-quality raw materials in animal feed is viewed critically. Mycotoxins, i.e. mould toxins that can develop in poor quality or improperly stored dry food, are also suspected of increasing the risk of cancer. A balanced, species-appropriate diet with high-quality processed, transparently labelled ingredients is therefore a significant preventative factor. Fresh ingredients, a balanced ratio of proteins, fats and carbohydrates and the avoidance of overfeeding are fundamental cornerstones of a healthy diet. There is also discussion as to whether certain nutrients such as omega-3 fatty acids, antioxidants or secondary plant substances have tumour-preventive properties - however, this has only been confirmed to a very limited extent and cannot be generalised.

Another important risk factor that is also being observed with increasing frequency in pets is obesity. Obesity leads to a variety of metabolic changes, including chronic inflammatory processes, impaired hormone regulation and increased oxidative stress - all factors that can also play a role in tumour development. Especially in the case of hormone-dependent tumours, such as mammary tumours or perianal adenomas, a connection with obesity seems plausible. However, a healthy body weight not only prevents cancer, but also reduces the risk of diabetes mellitus, joint diseases and cardiovascular problems, which represent a considerable burden, especially in older animals. Regular weight monitoring, needs-based feeding and the promotion of an active lifestyle are therefore essential measures in preventive healthcare.

Exercise not only contributes to weight control, but also has positive effects on the immune system, metabolism, cardiovascular fitness and behaviour. Animals that are regularly challenged physically and mentally show a higher overall resistance to stress, a better ability to regenerate and a more stable sense of well-being - all factors that play an indirect role in onco-prevention. Walks, phases of play, targeted exercise promotion in old age and species-appropriate husbandry are therefore essential not only in terms of quality of life, but also from a preventive medical perspective.

Finally, protection against known environmental carcinogens is a particularly relevant area. Numerous studies have shown that pets that regularly come into contact with tobacco smoke, pesticides, herbicides or industrial emissions have an increased risk of various types of tumours. Dogs in smoking households are more likely to develop nasal or lung tumours, while cats are more likely to ingest toxic substances by licking their pollutant-contaminated fur , which is associated with an increased risk of lymphoma, for example. Contact with treated green spaces, chemical cleaning agents or exhaust fumes can also have long-term health consequences. A conscious approach to chemical substances in the domestic environment and a critical examination of the environment for potential carcinogenic contamination are therefore of central importance.

In addition, UV radiation poses a serious risk in certain animals. Light-coloured or short-haired animals, especially white cats with pink-coloured noses and hairless ear rims, are particularly at risk of developing squamous cell carcinomas as a result of chronic sun exposure. Consistently avoiding direct exposure to the sun - especially at midday - and retreating to shady areas is a sensible preventative approach here. In some cases, the use of special sunscreens for animals can even be useful.

Overall, it is clear that promoting a healthy lifestyle is also a forward-looking and integral part of tumour prevention in pets. Diet, exercise, weight control and environmental protection form the basis of a holistic preventive strategy that can not only reduce the risk of tumours, but also make animals' lives healthier, more active and more enjoyable overall. Veterinary advice plays a key role in educating pet owners about these interrelationships, making personalised recommendations and promoting a culture of health that focuses not only on treatment, but above all on prevention.

9.3 Genetic screening in breeding animals

A particularly effective, but often underestimated lever in long-term tumour prevention lies in breeding control. Numerous oncological diseases in dogs and cats show a clear breed-specific accumulation, which indicates genetically fixed predispositions within certain populations. These patterns are not coincidental, but the expression of longstanding breeding practices in which external characteristics, temperament or performance criteria were in the foreground, while genetic predispositions - especially for complex diseases such as tumours - often went unnoticed or were only recognised too late. In a modern, health-oriented breeding strategy, it is therefore of central importance to identify genetic risks at an early stage, take targeted countermeasures and thus reduce the incidence of tumours in affected breeds in the long term.

Tumour diseases with a pronounced breed-specific prevalence include mast cell tumours in the Boxer, osteosarcomas in large breeds such as the Great Dane, Rottweiler or Irish Wolfhound as well as malignant lymphomas, which occur more frequently in Golden Retrievers, Labradors or Bernese Mountain Dogs. Histiocytic sarcomas also show an above-average prevalence in certain breeds, which indicates recessive or polygenic genetic variants. Such clinical pictures often occur at a relatively young age and are associated with high biological aggressiveness and limited treatment options. The targeted identification of predisposed breeding animals is therefore a key step towards reducing this disease burden in the herd as a whole.

Modern molecular genetic testing methods open up new possibilities in this context. Through targeted screening for known mutations or genetic risk factors, carrier animals can be identified even before clinical symptoms appear. Particularly in affected breeds where established genetic markers are already known - for example for certain forms of B-cell lymphoma in Golden Retrievers or for histiocytic sarcomas in Bernese Mountain Dogs - the targeted exclusion of such animals from breeding can make a significant contribution to reducing the incidence of the disease. The combination of genetic screening and careful breeding selection makes it possible to exclude not only affected animals but also asymptomatic gene carriers from further breeding and thus systematically reduce the spread of defective alleles within the population.

However, the implementation of this strategy requires a coordinated approach by all stakeholders involved. Breeding associations must be prepared to integrate genetic health criteria into their breeding regulations on a mandatory basis and establish participation in screening programmes as a compulsory component of a responsible breeding policy. Veterinarians take on an advisory, diagnostic and educational role by informing breeders about available test procedures, their significance and the consequences of the test results. Owners, for their part, bear responsibility by specifically supporting breeders who emphasise genetic diversity, health prevention and longevity - and consciously oppose suppliers who are dominated by aesthetic criteria or short-sighted interests.

In addition to the targeted exclusion of gene carriers, broader measures for genetic diversification within the breeds can also make a positive contribution. Narrow inbreeding coefficients, excessive line breeding or the repeated use of individual popular sires ("popular sire effect") not only increase the risk of recessive hereditary diseases, but also the genetic fixation of tumour-associated mutations. A structured breeding policy based on genetic diversity can mitigate this effect and improve the population's resilience to multifactorial diseases such as cancer.

In the long term, the integration of genetic health criteria into breeding practice not only keeps individual animals healthy, but also contributes to a sustainable reduction in tumour-related diseases in the population as a whole. This preventive effect unfolds over generations and is therefore a central component of forward-looking, responsible veterinary medicine. Breeding control is thus being transformed from a traditionally selective discipline into a strategic instrument of modern tumour prevention - supported by interdisciplinary cooperation, scientific transparency and a shared ethical self-image for the benefit of future generations of domestic animals.

9.4 Education and training of animal owners

An informed and educated pet owner is a key partner in the prevention of tumours. Many tumours could be detected at an earlier stage or prevented from occurring altogether if pet owners were informed about risk factors, early symptoms and preventive measures. Veterinarians should therefore proactively provide information about cancer and make suitable materials available - be it in the form of consultations, brochures, online information or lectures.

Particular attention should be paid to raising awareness of subtle changes. Early recognition of swellings, changes in skin areas, loss of appetite or unusual behaviour is only possible if the pet owner knows what to look out for. Dealing with unclear findings, the importance of regular follow-up care and the need for timely veterinary clarification should also be discussed.

Education also means countering myths and misconceptions - such as the alleged "cancer risk from vaccinations", the uncritical use of alternative remedies or exaggerated expectations of certain therapies. An objective, trusting dialogue strengthens the health literacy of the owners and makes a decisive contribution to successful prevention.

10. Research and future prospects in veterinary oncology

Veterinary oncology is a specialised field that is undergoing dynamic change. Technological innovations, molecular biological findings, new forms of therapy and increasing integration with human medicine are opening up perspectives that seemed unthinkable just a few decades ago. Veterinary medicine is no longer just a field of application for existing therapies, but is increasingly developing into an independent, research-driven scientific field. The future development of cancer therapy in pets will largely depend on the extent to which it is possible to transfer scientific findings into practice, strengthen interdisciplinary co-operation and at the same time meet the needs of animals, owners and society.

10.1 Current study situation and translational research status

The current study situation in veterinary oncology is characterised by a remarkable dynamism that is visible in both the breadth and depth of scientific research. In a field that has been overshadowed by human medical oncology for many years, there is now a clear tendency towards valorisation . Numerous veterinary colleges, university research institutions and privately organised pharmaceutical companies are increasingly investing in the development of new diagnostic procedures, therapeutic substances and individualised treatment concepts. This is accompanied by a clear professionalisation of the field, which is developing from a purely clinical discipline into a molecular biology-based, translationally oriented scientific discipline.

At the centre of this development is the so-called translational approach - a methodological concept that aims to translate fundamental findings from molecular biology, cell research and genetics into specific clinical applications. This principle makes it possible to bridge the gap between laboratory and clinic, between basic experimental research and everyday veterinary medicine. It is particularly noteworthy that veterinary oncology not only benefits from developments in human medicine, but is also increasingly recognised as an independent source of innovative therapeutic concepts.

A paradigmatic example of this successful translation is the research and application of tyrosine kinase inhibitors in canine mast cell tumours. These tumours are among the most common malignant skin neoplasms in dogs and in many cases have mutations in the so-called c-kit gene, which codes for a receptor tyrosine kinase. This mutation leads to a constitutive activation of the signalling pathway that promotes tumour growth. Drugs such as toceranib or masitinib, which were originally developed as part of human cancer research, have been successfully tested in veterinary studies on dogs with spontaneously occurring mast cell tumours and have been adopted in clinical practice. The high biological similarity of these spontaneous tumours to comparable human medical conditions makes dogs and cats particularly valuable models for the preclinical and clinical testing of new substances. In contrast to classical laboratory research, where tumours are artificially induced, these spontaneous neoplasms authentically reflect the complexity of real disease progression, genetic heterogeneity and immune interactions.

Veterinary research has also made significant progress in the field of immuno-oncology in recent years. The development of tumour vaccinology approaches, such as vaccines against malignant melanomas in dogs, marks a decisive step towards biologically individualised cancer therapies. These vaccines aim to specifically activate the animal's immune system against tumour antigens in order to generate a sustained and specific immune response. At the same time, immunomodulators are being researched that intervene in the interaction between the tumour and the immune system, for example by blocking immunosuppressive mechanisms or by strengthening cytotoxic reactions. Another innovative field is the use of autologous cell therapies, in which immunologically active cells of the patient - such as dendritic cells or T cells - are manipulated ex vivo and then re-administered in order to induce a targeted anti-tumour response.

These developments show that veterinary medicine is increasingly not only a co-user but also an active co-creator of innovative therapy concepts. The growing importance of domestic animals as model organisms for comparative oncology has led to veterinary research also attracting increasing attention in human medicine. In times in which personalised medicine, immunological procedures and molecular target structures form the standard of modern cancer therapy, veterinary oncology represents a highly relevant, practical and ethically justifiable field of research that makes an integral contribution to oncological innovation.

In addition, the increasing establishment of multi-centre study networks and standardised databases is an indicator of the professionalisation of veterinary oncology research. Interdisciplinary collaboration, structured study designs and the integration of clinical and molecular biological parameters now enable data quality that is internationally compatible. This not only increases the informative value of individual studies, but also creates the basis for evidence-based therapy recommendations that meet the requirements of modern veterinary medicine.

Overall, it can be said that veterinary oncological research is currently undergoing a phase of profound transformation. It is not only benefiting from advances in human medicine, but is also increasingly developing its own, animal-specific innovation paths. The close integration of basic research, clinical application and translational science is opening up a broad spectrum of therapeutic possibilities that could both improve the prognosis of animals suffering from cancer and make a valuable contribution to comparative oncology in the future.

10.2 Integration of AI, big data and molecular diagnostics

Digitalisation opens up completely new possibilities for veterinary oncology. Thanks to the integration of artificial intelligence and big data analyses, huge amounts of data from patient files, genetic analyses, imaging and therapy results can now be systematically evaluated and transferred into practice-relevant decision-making algorithms. This results in prognosis models that enable a more precise assessment of the course of the disease and generate individualised therapy suggestions.

Molecular diagnostics plays a key role in this context. By analysing tumour DNA, RNA expression profiles, epigenetics and protein markers, the biology of a tumour can be understood much better. The development of "liquid biopsies" - i.e. the detection of circulating tumour components in the blood - even opens up the possibility of a non-invasive, early and dynamically verifiable diagnosis in the future.

The combination with AI also leads to new standards in the field of imaging: Image analysis programmes recognise subtle changes earlier and more accurately than the human eye and can automatically quantify metastases or infiltrative growth, for example. These technical advances promise not only more objectivity, but also an improvement in the reproducibility of veterinary decisions.

10.3 Development of innovative therapeutic approaches

The ongoing development of new therapeutic approaches in veterinary oncology reflects the growing complexity and innovative power of this speciality. Parallel to the advances in diagnostics, the therapy options have also diversified and expanded in a remarkable way. In addition to traditional procedures such as surgery, radiotherapy and chemotherapy, modern, biologically orientated methods that target the cellular, genetic and molecular level are increasingly coming to the fore. These new strategies are not only aimed at directly combating tumours, but also at activating the body's own defence mechanisms, modulating the microenvironment and stabilising the oncological balance in the long term.

A particularly promising approach for the future is cell-based therapy, in which immune cells are used specifically to fight tumours. In human medicine, so-called CAR-T cells - genetically modified T lymphocytes equipped with chimeric antigen receptors - have already achieved groundbreaking success in certain forms of leukaemia and lymphoma. Initial studies are also underway in veterinary research in which this technique is being applied to spontaneous tumours in dogs and cats. The aim is to activate the patient's own immune cells outside the body, genetically reprogramme them and then reintroduce them in order to generate a targeted immune response against the tumour cells. Autologous cell therapy, which does not necessarily involve genetic modifications, but instead stimulates immune cells - such as dendritic cells or T cells - through antigen contact and re-infuses them into the animal, is considered particularly promising. This individualised form of therapy has the advantage that it can be tailored precisely to the immunological profile of the individual animal and is potentially highly effective and well tolerated.

Alongside these cell-based procedures, intensive research is also being conducted into the combination of different forms of therapy as part of multimodal protocols. Numerous studies have shown that the combination of surgical tumour removal, subsequent immunotherapy and supplementary radiotherapy often leads to better results than each individual measure on its own. The synergy effects of these integrated treatment concepts are based on the fact that different points of attack can be used, systemic spreading foci can be controlled and the immunological recognition of tumour cells can be improved. Such strategies are supported by new drug delivery technologies: liposomal carrier systems enable the targeted release of active substances at the site of action, nanotechnological vehicles improve the bioavailability of poorly soluble substances and locally applicable drug depots enable sustained, minimally invasive drug release with a reduced side effect profile.

Another much-noticed trend is the development of dietary interventions that can be used not only as an adjunct to therapy, but also as an independent measure to influence tumour metabolism . The basis of these concepts is the realisation that tumour cells often exhibit altered energy production - such as increased glycolysis even under oxygen conditions ("Warburg effect") - and therefore react particularly sensitively to certain nutrients. Cancer diets that are low in carbohydrates and high in fat, for example, are intended to exploit these metabolic characteristics in order to inhibit the growth of tumour cells and strengthen healthy tissue. Although these approaches appear promising, the study situation in veterinary medicine is not yet standardised, meaning that their use should always be critically examined and individually adapted.

In addition, phytomedicinal substances are increasingly being used in oncological research. Natural substances such as curcumin, artemisinin or resveratrol show antitumour, anti-inflammatory and antioxidant properties in vitro and in animal studies. However, their exact mode of action, optimal dosage and clinical relevance in dogs and cats are the subject of ongoing research, as the results to date are sometimes contradictory and standardised preparations are hardly available to date. Nevertheless, these substances offer interesting potential as complementary therapy components, particularly in the context of integrative treatment concepts that combine elements of conventional medicine and naturopathy.

Overall, it can be said that the treatment of tumour diseases in pets is currently entering a new phase characterised by biological precision, individual adaptation and technological innovation. The future of veterinary oncology no longer lies exclusively in the aggressive fight against tumours, but increasingly in the intelligent modulation of biological processes, the strengthening of the body's own defence systems and the targeted combination of differently effective therapeutic pillars. This development not only opens up new therapeutic possibilities, but also requires a rethink in diagnostics, planning and communication - towards a holistic, scientifically based and individually orientated veterinary oncology.

10.4 Interdisciplinary collaboration with human medicine

One particularly dynamic area is the increasing interlinking of human and veterinary oncology. This interdisciplinary cooperation follows the so-called One Health approach, which assumes that human and animal health are closely linked. Dogs and cats with spontaneous tumours are now regarded as valuable models for the development of new therapies in humans, particularly because they have similar environmental conditions, immune responses and disease progression.

Veterinarians, human physicians, pharmacologists, molecular biologists and bioinformaticians work together in large international research networks to develop new drugs, vaccines and diagnostic procedures. Veterinary clinics act not only as treatment centres, but increasingly also as research locations with clinical studies, biobank programmes and molecular genetic databases.

For veterinary medicine, this opens up the opportunity to participate directly in medical innovation - not only as a recipient of human medical developments, but also as an active contributor. Involvement in interdisciplinary projects strengthens the quality of veterinary care, promotes scientific progress and contributes to the social recognition of veterinary medicine as an independent research discipline.

11. Legal and insurance-related framework conditions

The diagnosis and treatment of cancer in pets not only raises medical and ethical questions, but also concerns a number of legal and insurance-related aspects. These include the duty to inform and obtain consent from pet owners, the civil liability of veterinarians, billing and cost coverage by pet health insurance companies as well as the documentation and, in exceptional cases, the obligation to report certain diseases. In practice, these issues often only become virulent when complications, treatment cancellations or misunderstandings occur. It is therefore all the more important that veterinarians and animal owners are well informed about the legal framework.

11.1 Liability issues in connection with diagnostics and therapy

The civil liability of veterinarians is regulated differently internationally, but has common features in many legal systems. In Germany, Austria and Switzerland, animals are legally regarded as "objects of a special kind" or "movable objects with special protection status". As a result, veterinary treatment is generally provided in accordance with the rules on services that are to be provided properly and professionally, without any success - in the sense of a cure or complete recovery - being owed. The veterinarian is therefore only liable for errors in the execution of the treatment

(treatment errors), but not for its outcome, provided that the duty of care has been observed.

In France, the legal categorisation of animals has been more differentiated since the reform of the Civil Code in 2015. Pursuant to *Article 515-14 of the Civil Code*, animals are no longer considered exclusively as objects, but as "sentient beings" (êtres *vivants doués de sensibilité*), although they are still subject to substantive law unless more specific provisions exist. The civil liability of the veterinarian is based on the general professional liability in accordance with *the Code de la santé publique* and the *Code civil*. Here, too, there is a duty to perform the treatment professionally, but not to cure. However, incorrect diagnoses, inadequate information or improper treatment can give rise to tortious or contractual liability.

In Spain, animals are still formally regarded as property (*bienes muebles*) under the Civil Code (*Código Civil*), although there has recently been a recognisable trend towards reform in terms of improved animal welfare. Since the law reform 17/2021 of December 2021, animals have been granted special protection status as "sentient beings". With regard to veterinary liability, the contractual relationship is usually interpreted as a service contract, similar to that in Germany. The veterinarian owes a professionally correct service, but not a successful treatment. The basis for liability can result from breach of contract (*incumplimiento contractual*) or from unauthorised action (*responsabilidad extracontractual*).

In Italy, the *Codice Civile* continues to regard animals as movable property (*bene mobile*), although there is increasing normative and judicial recognition of animals as fellow creatures with a special right to protection. Veterinary liability is based on the service contract in accordance with *Art. 2222 ff. Codice Civile*. Here too, the following applies: The veterinarian is not liable for the failure of the treatment, but only for incorrect execution, for example due to lack of care, incorrect diagnosis or improper aftercare. In addition, tortious liability under *Art. 2043 Codice Civile* may also be considered in the event of serious breaches of duty.

In Anglo-American jurisdictions, particularly in the United Kingdom and the United States, animals are also treated as *property*. Veterinary liability there is typically based on *contract law* and *tort law*. Veterinarians are obliged to act with the due care and expertise expected of a "reasonably competent practitioner" . There is no obligation to provide a cure here either. However, in cases of proven *negligence*, failure to provide information or incorrect treatment, civil liability may exist. In the USA, *informed consent* - i.e. the comprehensive explanation of risks and alternatives to the animal owner - is also a central aspect in the assessment of liability. In individual cases, liability can also include compensation for emotional distress or immaterial damage, although this is handled with varying degrees of rigour depending on the state.

In the field of oncology, there are increased requirements for information about risks, side effects and prospects of success. If, for example, chemotherapy leads to serious side effects or complications as a result of a surgical procedure, the question arises as to whether the vet has provided thorough information, documented it correctly and acted in accordance with veterinary standards. An incorrect diagnosis, inadequate therapy monitoring or the wrong choice of medication can have consequences under liability law if the animal was harmed as a result and a breach of duty of care can be proven.

Situations in which a decision not to treat is accompanied by the death of the animal or a therapy was continued although a palliative medical approach would have been more appropriate are particularly delicate. The question of reasonableness and ethical considerations also becomes relevant here, which makes sound medical and legally secure communication with the pet owner all the more urgent.

11.2 Role of veterinary health insurance for oncological diseases

Pet health insurance has become considerably more important in recent years, particularly in the area of costly diagnostics and long-term therapy. Many providers cover the costs of operations, medication, imaging procedures and even chemotherapy - but only if the insured benefits are not limited by specific exclusions. Tumour diseases are explicitly named as insured events in some policies, while in others they are partially or completely excluded from the scope of benefits by blanket exclusions.

It is therefore essential for pet owners to check the conditions carefully before taking out insurance. These include waiting periods, upper limits per year or treatment, deductibles and restrictions for pre-existing conditions or genetically predisposed breeds. If a tumour has already been diagnosed, it is generally no longer possible to take out a new insurance policy at , which means that taking precautions at an early stage can also be financially worthwhile.

For veterinarians, working with insurance companies means an additional administrative task. At the same time, however, it can also have a positive influence on treatment decisions, as financial security provides greater scope for high-quality treatments. Transparent communication about expected costs, insurance benefit limits and possible follow-up treatments is essential in order to avoid misunderstandings and frustration on the part of owners.

11.3 Duty to inform and consent of owners

Informing the animal owner about the planned therapy, its prospects of success, risks, side effects and alternatives is not only a medical-ethical obligation, but also a legally protected component of the treatment. Only if the animal owner consents to the measure on the basis of comprehensive information is the intervention legally permissible.

Information is often complex, particularly in the case of oncological treatments, as the balance between benefit and risk is not always clear. The vet must explain what diagnostic steps are necessary, what therapeutic options are available, what burdens will be placed on the animal and how high the costs are likely to be. The possibility of discontinuing treatment, the importance of quality of life and the decision on palliative care or euthanasia should also be discussed in advance.

11.4 Documentation and reporting obligations for certain tumours

The documentation of diagnostics, therapy and follow-up is a central element of veterinary due diligence. It serves the traceability of medical decisions, legal self-protection, quality assurance and the possibility of analysing disease progression for scientific purposes. Detailed documentation of the clinical picture, diagnostic steps, laboratory findings, imaging, treatment planning, course of medication and communication with the owner is essential, particularly in the case of complex diseases such as cancer.

A general obligation to report tumour diseases does not yet exist in most European countries. However, there are exceptions: For example, certain viral tumours (such as diseases caused by papillomaviruses or leukosis viruses) are subject to mandatory reporting in individual cases, for example in the livestock sector or in cross-border animal traffic. Voluntary or project-related reporting obligations may also apply to clinical studies, participation in biobanks or collaboration with oncological research databases.

The digitalisation of veterinary practices offers great opportunities here: electronic patient files, standardised diagnostic documentation and digital interfaces to research institutions can improve the quality of documentation and contribute to better recording of oncological diseases in livestock in the long term.

12. Future prospects and new healing methods

The treatment of cancer in pets is on the threshold of a fundamental change. New scientific findings from molecular biology, cell research, genetics, medical technology and immunology are not only opening up innovative therapeutic approaches, but are also changing our understanding of tumour biology and disease progression. What was considered incurable a few decades ago can now be controlled in many cases, and a purely palliative veterinary medicine is increasingly developing into a curative and individualised oncology. The future of cancer treatment in pets will be characterised by integration, precision and biological depth.

A central element of this development is the increasing individualisation of therapies. Standardised protocols, which are applied regardless of the individual tumour profile, are being replaced by targeted treatment based on molecular characteristics. The genetic analysis of tumour tissue - also known as tumour profiling - enables the identification of mutation-specific targets. This allows targeted drugs to be administered that only affect tumour cells without damaging healthy tissue. Such approaches have already been successfully implemented in clinical practice for mast cell tumours and will be used for a large number of other tumour types in the future.

Another promising area is immuno-oncology. Here, the body's own immune system is activated or specifically directed to recognise and destroy tumour cells. While classic immunostimulation is already being used in the form of tumour vaccines and immunomodulators, the scientific focus is increasingly turning to more complex strategies such as checkpoint inhibitors, dendritic cell therapies or CAR-T cells. Initial studies are showing positive results, particularly in dogs with malignant lymphomas or melanomas, although many of these methods are still at an experimental stage.

Gene therapy is also becoming increasingly important. Targeted modification of genetic information within the tumour cells or the surrounding tissue is intended to stop growth processes, reactivate apoptosis mechanisms or switch off resistance mechanisms. The difficulty so far lies in the precise control and safe application of these techniques, but advances in the field of viral vectors and nanotechnology make an application in veterinary oncology plausible in the near future.

Regenerative medicine offers complementary and partially overlapping approaches. Stem cell-based procedures are increasingly being investigated not only to support damaged tissue after intensive therapy, but also to modulate immune responses or as carriers of regenerative growth factors. These technologies potentially enable a combination of tumour reduction and tissue healing, which is particularly relevant for highly invasive or surgically stressful tumour forms.

Technological innovations such as robotics, 3D printing, personalised implants and intraoperative navigation could make surgical procedures more precise, tissue-friendly and easier to control in the future. The combination of image-guided surgical technology with mechanical assistance opens up a new dimension of feasibility, particularly for difficult-to-access tumours in the cranial region, spine or pelvic area.

In addition to therapy, the approaches to early detection and progression monitoring are also changing. The use of liquid biopsies, i.e. the analysis of circulating tumour DNA in the blood, promises early diagnosis, the detection of minimal residual disease after therapy and the real-time monitoring of resistance developments. The combination of imaging with artificial intelligence - for the automated detection of metastases, for example - will also play a decisive role in oncological monitoring in the future.

The digitalisation of veterinary medicine as a whole will also have a decisive impact on the future of oncology. Cloud-based patient records, interactive treatment protocols, AI-supported decision trees and globally networked research databases will significantly improve the quality, consistency and evidence-based nature of treatment. Interdisciplinary collaboration in particular - for example between pathologists, internists, surgeons and oncologists - can be made more efficient, more timely and more location-independent using digital tools.

Finally, the change in society's relationship with pets is also pointing the way to the future. The willingness of many owners to utilise complex and cost-intensive therapies is growing steadily. This creates the basis for investment in new procedures, the expansion of specialist animal oncology centres and the establishment of clinical study structures within veterinary medicine. At the same time, however, there is also a need for an ethical discussion on how far treatment can go, when quality of life should take precedence over prolonging life and what standards should apply to animal welfare in the age of high technology.

Overall, it can be said that the future of cancer therapy in pets will be characterised by profound scientific, technological and social changes. The boundaries between curative and palliative medicine, between research and practice, between veterinary and human oncology are becoming increasingly blurred. This opens up new opportunities - but also new responsibilities. Veterinary medicine is therefore faced with the task of not only further developing its oncological possibilities, but also using them wisely, responsibly and with empathy.

13. Concluding remarks

Dealing with cancer in pets inevitably leads to the interface between modern medical science, practical veterinary medicine, ethical awareness and the emotional bond between humans and animals. It is therefore more than just a technical or diagnostic challenge - it is an expression of an attitude that takes animal life seriously in its vulnerability, but also in its dignity.

In the course of this work, it became clear that veterinary oncology is no longer limited to the detection and treatment of individual tumour forms, but has grown into an independent, interdisciplinary field. It combines basic biological research with highly developed imaging, surgical precision, drug diversity and immunological sophistication. At the same time, it requires a deep understanding of the individual progression, the nature of the animal, the resilience of the owners and the dynamics of a disease that cannot be controlled schematically.

The findings from tumour biology and molecular veterinary medicine have taught us that cancer is not a monolithic process, but rather a multi-layered process made up of genetic, epigenetic, hormonal and environmental factors. The diversity of clinical manifestations reflects this complexity, as do the different responses to therapeutic interventions. No two tumours are the same, and no treatment can be based solely on statistics - it must always be geared to the specific case, the specific animal, its behaviour and its biography.

At the same time, it became clear that despite all the advances in diagnostics and therapy, the quality of life of the animal must always be at the centre of attention. Veterinary oncology must not become an end in itself of ever more complex medicine, but must always measure its methods by whether they can alleviate suffering, preserve dignity and maintain joie de vivre. This attitude requires a new balance between technical possibilities and animal ethical responsibility - a balance that does not result from textbooks, but from experience, empathy and honest dialogue with the animal owner.

The future of veterinary oncology lies in integration: the integration of natural science and clinical practice, of diagnostics and therapy, of standardisation and individualisation, of research and compassion. It lies in the willingness to embrace new knowledge, but not to implement it without reflection; in the ability to offer hope without making false promises; and in the wisdom to understand the end of a life not as a defeat, but as part of care.

Cancer treatment in pets will therefore continue to be a reflection of our medical progress and our moral stance. Its quality will not only be measured by its technical brilliance, but also by the humanity with which it is practised. With this in mind, this book is intended not only to impart knowledge, but also to stimulate reflection - about the animal as a patient, about veterinary medicine as a vocation and about pet owners as part of a community of responsibility that extends far beyond medical treatment.

14. Bibliography

Alvarez, F. J., & Kisseberth, W. C. (2021). *Cancer chemotherapy in small animal practice* (2nd ed.). Wiley-Blackwell.

Boston, S. E., & Ehrhart, N. P. (Eds.). (2020). *Decision making in small animal oncology*. John Wiley & Sons.

Chand Khanna, C., Lindblad-Toh, K., Vail, D. M., & London, C. A. (2020). The dog as a cancer model. *Nature Reviews Cancer*, 20(7), 543-560. https://doi.org/10.1038/s41568-020-0271-3

Cooper, T. L., & Burton, J. H. (2019). Advances in veterinary oncology. *Veterinary Clinics of North America: Small Animal Practice*, 49(5), 819-834. https://doi.org/10.1016/j.cvsm.2019.05.005

Dobson, J. M., Samuel, S., Milstein, H., Rogers, K., & Wood, J. L. N. (2002). Canine neoplasia in the UK: Estimates of incidence rates from a population of insured dogs. *Journal of Small Animal Practice*, 43(6), 240-246. https://doi.org/10.1111/j.1748-5827.2002.tb00066.x

Etienne, C., Marescaux, L., & Fournet, A. (2021). Ethics of palliative care in veterinary medicine. *Animals*, 11(5), 1428. https://doi.org/10.3390/ani11051428

Fleming, J. M., Creevy, K. E., & Promislow, D. E. L. (2011). Mortality in North American dogs from 1984 to 2004: An investigation into age-, size-, and breed-related causes of death. *Journal of Veterinary Internal Medicine*, 25(2), 187-198. https://doi.org/10.1111/j.1939-1676.2011.0695.x

Foster, R. A., & Withrow, S. J. (2020). *Withrow and MacEwen's small animal clinical oncology* (6th ed.). Elsevier.

Gieger, T. L. (2016). Alimentary lymphoma in cats and dogs. *Veterinary Clinics: Small Animal Practice*, 46(1), 89-112. https://doi.org/10.1016/j.cvsm.2015.09.006

Hahn, K. A., Richardson, R. C., Hahn, E. A., & Chrisman, C. L. (1994). Diagnostic and therapeutic advances in veterinary oncology. *Journal of the American Veterinary Medical Association*, 204(8), 1162-1165.

Henry, C. J. (2017). Cancer management in small animal practice. *Veterinary Clinics of North America: Small Animal Practice*, 47(5), 847-862. https://doi.org/10.1016/j.cvsm.2017.04.007

Knapp, D. W., Glickman, N. W., DeNicola, D. B., Bonney, P. L., Lin, T. L., & Glickman, L. T. (2000). Naturally-occurring canine transitional cell carcinoma of the urinary bladder: A relevant model of human invasive bladder cancer. *Urologic Oncology*, 5(2), 47-59. https://doi.org/10.1016/S1078-1439(99)00023-3

Marconato, L., & Zini, E. (2014). *Veterinary oncology: Clinical aspects and therapeutic perspectives*. Springer.

Mellanby, R. J., & Herrtage, M. E. (2022). *Veterinary medicine: A textbook of the diseases of cattle, horses, sheep, pigs and goats* (12th ed.). Elsevier.

Modiano, J. F., Breen, M., Burnett, R. C., Parker, H. G., Inusah, S., Thomas, R., Avery, P. R., Avery, A. C., & Lindblad-Toh, K. (2005). Distinct B-cell and T-cell lymphoproliferative disease prevalence among dog breeds indicates heritable risk. *Cancer Research*, 65(13), 5654-5661. https://doi.org/10.1158/0008-5472.CAN-04-4613

Moore, A. S., & Ruple, A. (2022). Translational oncology in veterinary medicine. *Veterinary Sciences*, 9(3), 129. https://doi.org/10.3390/vetsci9030129

Polton, G. A., Brearley, M. J., Powell, S. M., & White, R. A. S. (2005). Impact of primary tumour stage on survival after surgery for canine mammary carcinoma. *Journal of Small Animal Practice*, 46(9), 429-434. https://doi.org/10.1111/j.1748-5827.2005.tb00272.x

Sørensen, M. A., & Kristensen, A. T. (2015). The future of veterinary oncology: Genomics and beyond. *Veterinary Journal*, 205(2), 125-132. https://doi.org/10.1016/j.tvjl.2015.04.006

Vail, D. M., Thamm, D. H., & Liptak, J. M. (Eds.). (2020). *Withrow & MacEwen's small animal clinical oncology* (6th ed.). Elsevier.

Von Euler, H., & Egenvall, A. (2016). The Swedish veterinary cancer registry: A continuous registration of tumours in companion animals. *European Journal of Comparative Oncology*, 1(3), 81-86. https://doi.org/10.1016/j.ejco.2016.05.004

Withrow, S. J., Vail, D. M., & Page, R. L. (2013). *Withrow and MacEwen's small animal clinical oncology* (5th ed.). Elsevier.